Surgical Critical Care Vivas

For my wife, Pauline Cornelia O'Keeffe

Surgical Critical Care Vivas

Mazyar Kanani BSc (Hons) MBBS (Hons) MRCS (Eng)

British Heart Foundation
Paediatric Cardiothoracic Clinical Research Fellow
Cardiac Unit
Great Ormond Street Hospital
London, UK

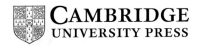

CAMBRIDGE
UNIVERSITY PRESS

CAMBRIDGE UNIVERSITY PRESS
Cambridge, New York, Melbourne, Madrid, Cape Town, Singapore, São Paulo, Delhi

Cambridge University Press
The Edinburgh Building, Cambridge CB2 8RU, UK

Published in the United States of America by Cambridge University Press, New York

www.cambridge.org
Information on this title: www.cambridge.org/9780521681537

First published 2003
Sixth printing 2008

Printed in the United Kingdom at the University Press, Cambridge

A catalogue record for this publication is available from the British Library

ISBN 978-0-521-68153-7 paperback

CONTENTS

CONTENTS

LIST OF ABBREVIATIONS

ACTH	Adrenocorticotropic hormone
ADH	Anti diuretic hormone
ADP	Adenosine diphosphate
ALI	Acute lung injury
AMP	Adenosine monophosphate
APTT	Activated partial thromboplastin time
ARDS	Acute respiratory distress syndrome
ATLS	Advance trauma life support
ATN	Acute tubular necrosis
ATP	Adenosine triphosphate
ATPase	Adenosine triphosphatase
AV	Atrioventricular
BBB	Blood-brain barrier
2,3 BPG	2,3 Bisphosphoglycerate
CAPD	Citrate, Adenine, Phosphate, and Dextrose
cGMP	Cyclic guanosine monophosphate
CMV	Cytomegalovirus
CO	Cardiac output
COPD	Chronic obstructive pulmonary disease
CPAP	Continuous positive airway pressure
CSF	Cerebrospinal fluid
CVP	Central venous pressure
CXR	Chest radiograph
DIC	Disseminated Intravascular Coagulation
DKA	Diabetic ketoacidosis
DPL	Diagnostic peritoneal lavage
DVT	Deep venous thrombosis
ECF	Extracellular fluid
ECG	Electrocardiogram
ELISA	Enzyme linked immunosorbent assay
ESR	Erythrocyte sedimentation rate
FFA	Free fatty acids
FFP	Fresh frozen plasma
FiO$_2$	Fraction of inspired oxygen

FRC	Functional residual capacity
GCS	Glasgow coma score
GFR	Glomerular filtration rate
HITS	Heparin-induced thrombocytopenia syndrome
HIV	Human immunodeficiency virus
HLA	Human leucocyte antigen
HMSO	Her Majesty's Stationery Office
HRT	Hormone replacement therapy
I:E RATIO	Inspiratory:Expiratory ratio
ICF	Intracellular fluid
ICP	Intracranial pressure
IgA	Immunoglobulin A
IL	Interleukin
IMV	Intermittent mandatory ventilation
INR	International normalised ratio
IPPV	Intermittent positive pressure ventilation
ITU	Intensive therapy unit
JVP	Jugular venous pulse/pressure
MAP	Mean arterial pressure
MI	Myocardial infarction
MODS	Multi-Organ dysfunction syndrome
MPAP	Mean pulmonary artery pressure
MRI	Magnetic resonance imaging
MRSA	Methicillin resistant *Staph. aureus*
NG	Nasogastric
NJ	Nasojejunal
NSAIDs	Non-steroidal anti-inflammatory drugs
PA	Pulmonary artery
PAF	Platelet activating factor
PAOP	Pulmonary artery occlusion pressure
PCA	Patient-controlled analgesia
PCC	Prothrombin complex concentrate
PE	Pulmonary embolus
PEEP	Positive end-expiratory pressure
PSV	Pressure support ventilation
PTH	Parathormone
PVR	Pulmonary vascular resistance

RAA	Renin–angiotensin–aldosterone
SAMG	Saline, Adenine, Mannitol, and Glucose
SaO_2	Arterial oxygen saturation
SIADH	Syndrome of inappropriate ADH
SIMV	Synchronised intermittent mandatory ventilation
SIRS	Systemic inflammatory response syndrome
SLE	Systemic lupus erythmatosus
SVC	Superior caval vein
SvO_2	Mixed venous oxygen saturation
SVR	Systemic vascular resistance
SVT	Supra-ventricular tacycardia
TB	Tuberculosis
TNF	Tumour necrosis factor
TPN	Parenteral nutrition
TT	Thrombin time
TURP	Trans-urethral resection of the prostate
V/Q RATIO	Ventilation/perfusion ratio
VA	Alveolar ventilation
VSD	Ventricular septal defect

ACKNOWLEDGEMENTS

This project would not have been possible without the unfailing support and encouragement of Miss Marjan Jahangiri, Consultant Cardiac Surgeon to St George's Hospital, London. It is also a pleasure to acknowledge Gavin Smith and Gill Clark, publishers at GMM, whose enthusiasm from the outset made all the difference.

ACKNOWLEDGEMENTS

ABDOMINAL TRAUMA: INVESTIGATIONS

What are the two major types of abdominal trauma?

The two types of injury are blunt and penetrating. The abdomen may be considered as being composed of five parts:

- *Abdominal wall:* front and back

- *Subcostal portion:* containing the stomach, liver, spleen and lesser sac

- *Pelvic portion:* containing the rectum, internal genitalia and iliac vessels

- *Intraperitoneal portion* in between the above: containing the small and large bowel

- *Retroperitoneum:* containing the kidneys, urinary tract, great vessels, pancreas and the rest of the colon

Which abdominal organs are most commonly injured?

The three most commonly injured organs are the liver, spleen and kidneys.

How may suspected injuries be investigated?

The initial investigations performed to assess the abdomen as a whole are

- *Plain radiography:* also assesses the bony pelvis

- *Ultrasound:* particularly good for the presence of free fluid in the abdomen, or haematoma around solid organs. There is a 10% risk of missing a significant injury

- *Diagnostic peritoneal lavage (DPL):* this is 98% sensitive for intra-peritoneal bleeding

- *CT scanning:* this can be used if the results of the DPL are equivocal, and may also be performed at the same time as a brain scan. Very good for retroperitoneal injury, less so for hollow viscus injury such as the bowel

▼ 1

Under which circumstances would you perform a diagnostic peritoneal lavage (DPL)?

Some of the indications are

- A suspicion of abdominal trauma on clinical examination
- Unexplained hypotension: with the abdomen being the source of occult haemorrhage
- Equivocal abdominal examination because of head injury and reduced level of consciousness
- The presence of a wound that has traversed the abdominal wall, but there is no indication for immediate laparotomy, e.g. a stab wound in a stable patient

When is DPL contraindicated?

The most important contraindication for DPL is in the situation which calls for mandatory laparotomy, e.g. frank peritonitis following trauma, abdominal gunshot injury or a hypotensive patient with abdominal distension.

How is DPL most commonly performed?

Performance of a DPL by the open method

- Requires an aseptic technique
- The abdomen is decompressed by insertion of a urinary catheter and nasogastric tube
- Local anaesthetic is administered to the subumbilical area in the mid-line
- An incision is made over this point. If a pelvic fracture is suspected, then a supraumbilical incision is made to prevent haematoma disruption
- Dissection is performed down to the peritoneum and the cannula is inserted under direct vision, guiding it towards the pelvis
- One litre of warmed saline is infused. Tilting and gently rolling the patient helps distribution
- The bag of saline can be left on the floor to siphon off the sample fluid from the abdomen

What are the positive criteria with DPL?

- Lavage fluid appears in the chest drain or urinary catheter
- Frank blood on entering the abdomen
- Presence of bile or faeces
- Red cell count of $>100,000/\mu l$
- White cell count of $>500/\mu l$
- Amylase of $>175\,U/ml$

A

ACCESSING THE THORAX

In which major ways may the thorax be accessed?

- Percutaneous methods
  - *Needle thoracostomy:* to drain fluid, air or for biopsy of tissue
  - *Tube thoracostomy ('chest drain'):* for drainage of air or fluid
  - *Thoracoscopic surgery:* permits procedures such as lung/pleural biopsy, lobectomy, pleurodesis, pleurectomy, sympathectomy, pericardiocentesis and pericardial window
- Thoracotomy
  - *Median sternotomy:* from the top of the manubrium at the jugular notch, passing longitudinally through the sternum to the xiphisternum. It permits access to the pericardium, great vessels, and both hemithoraces
  - *Posterolateral thoracotomy:* the most common approach in thoracic surgery. The incision runs from a point mid-way between the medial scapular edge and the thoracic spine, following a curve that runs 2 cm below the inferior scapular angle, to the mid-point of the axilla
  - *Anterior thoracotomy:* from the sternal edge, curving laterally along the intercostal space below the nipple to the axilla. It allows lung, pericardial and lung access, and also to lymph nodes in the aorto-pulmonary window
  - *Posterior thoracotomy:* the line of the incision is similar to that of a posterolateral thoracotomy, but starts at a more posterior point, encroaching on to the trapezius and erector spinae muscles. It allows access to the lung and great vessels for some paediatric cardiac procedures
  - *Bilateral anterior sternotomy ('clamshell' incision):* this incision runs from below one nipple to the contralateral side, dividing the body of the sternum in-between. It permits emergency access to the

pericardium and simultaneous exposure of both pleural cavities

- **■** *Thoraco-laparotomy:* the incision runs like that of a posterolateral thoracotomy, but continues anteriorly to cross the costal margin at the junction of the sixth and seventh ribs. The line runs for another 5 cm into the abdominal wall. It is extended inferiorly as a para-median or mid-line laparotomy. It permits access to posterior mediastinal structures, such as the aorta or oesophagus as they run into the abdomen

- Mediastinoscopy: the incision runs across the anterior neck, two fingers-breadth above the jugular notch. Allows access to the sub-carinal lymph nodes for disease diagnosis and staging

Which important piece of anaesthetic equipment is required for thoracotomy, and why?

The double-lumen endobronchial tube. This permits the use of one-lung anaesthesia where one lung may be collapsed and inflated at will for the purposes of surgery. This is particularly important for thoracoscopy where one lung has to be collapsed to permit the safe passage of the instruments through the thoracic wall.

What is the important pre-requisite to closure of all thoracotomies?

Chest drain insertion. Post cardiac surgery, one or two drains may be inserted into the mediastinum/posterior peri-cardium, exiting through the skin subcostally. Other drains are placed into any opened pleural space, e.g. during internal mammary artery harvest. After thoracotomy, one apical and one basal chest drain may be placed, both exiting sub-costally.

Briefly mention some important local complications of thoracotomy.

Wound complications
- Early:
  - **■** Immediate dehiscence from poor technique

- Haematoma formation
- Poor pain control leading to atelectasis, retention of secretions, hypoxia and infection
- Intermediate:
  - Infection, leading to wound dehiscence
- Late:
  - Post-thoracotomy neuralgia

Pulmonary complications

- Early:
  - *Air leak:* seen as continuous bubbling from the drains when placed on suction. May be due to parenchymal injury or a leak from the suture-line of a bronchial stump
  - *Bleeding:* producing haemothorax. May be from the raw parenchymal surface, or from a larger vessel
- Intermediate:
  - *Pneumonia:* can lead to a lung abscess
  - *Pulmonary oedema:* seen particularly in the contralateral lung following pneumonectomy. May also occur following re-expansion of a chronically collapsed or compressed lung from effusion
- Late:
  - Chronic broncho-pleural fistula
  - Empyema

ACID-BASE

Define the pH.
The pH is $-\log_{10}[H^+]$.

What is the pH of blood?
7.36–7.44.

Where does the acid load (H^+) in the body come from?
Most of the H^+ in the body comes from CO_2 generated from metabolism. This enters solution, forming carbonic acid through a reaction mediated by the enzyme carbonic anhydrase.

$$CO_2 + H_2O \rightleftharpoons H_2CO_3 \rightleftharpoons H^+ + HCO_3^-$$

Acid is also generated by
- Metabolism of the sulphur-containing amino acids cysteine and methionine
- Anaerobic metabolism, generating lactic acid
- Generation of the ketone bodies acetone, acetoacetate and β-hydroxybutyrate

What are the main buffer systems in the intravascular, interstitial and intracellular compartments?
In the plasma the main systems are
- The bicarbonate system
- The phosphate system ($HPO_4^{2-} + H^+ \rightleftharpoons H_2PO_4^-$)
- Plasma proteins
- Globin component of haemoglobin

Interstitial: the bicarbonate system
Intracellular: cytoplasmic proteins

What does the Henderson–Hasselbalch equation describe, and how is it derived?
This equation, which may be applied to any buffer system, defines the relationship between dissociated and undissociated

acids and bases. It is used mainly to describe the equilibrium of the bicarbonate system.

$$CO_2 + H_2O \rightleftharpoons H_2CO_3 \rightleftharpoons H^+ + HCO_3^-$$

The dissociation constant,

$$K = \frac{[H^+][HCO_3^-]}{[H_2CO_3]}$$

Therefore

$$[H^+] = K\frac{[H_2CO_3]}{[HCO_3^-]}$$

Taking the log

$$\log[H^+] = \log K + \log\frac{[H_2CO_3]}{[HCO_3^-]}$$

Taking the negative log, which expresses the pH, and where $-\log K$ is the pK

$$pH = pK - \log\frac{[H_2CO_3]}{[HCO_3^-]}$$

Invert the term to remove the minus sign

$$pH = pK + \log\frac{[HCO_3^-]}{[H_2CO_3]}$$

The $[H_2CO_3]$ may be expressed as $pCO_2 \times 0.23$, where 0.23 is the solubility coefficient of CO_2 (when the pCO_2 is in kPa).

The pK is equal to 6.1.

Thus,

$$pH = 6.1 + \log\frac{[HCO_3^-]}{pCO_2 \times 0.23}.$$

Which organ systems are involved in regulating acid–base balance?

The main organ systems involved in regulating acid–base balance are

▼

- *Respiratory system:* this controls the pCO_2 through alterations in alveolar ventilation. Carbon dioxide indirectly stimulates central chemoceptors (found in the ventro-lateral surface of the medulla oblongata) through H^+ released when it crosses the blood–brain barrier (BBB) and dissolves in the cerebrospinal fluid (CSF)

- *Kidney:* this controls the $[HCO_3^-]$, and is important for long term control and compensation of acid–base disturbances

- *Blood:* through buffering by plasma proteins and haemoglobin

- *Bone:* H^+ may exchange with cations from bone mineral. There is also carbonate in bone that can be used to support plasma HCO_3^- levels

- *Liver:* this may generate HCO_3^- and NH_4^+ (ammonia) by glutamine metabolism. In the kidney tubules, ammonia excretion generates more bicarbonate

How does the kidney absorb bicarbonate?

There are three main methods by which the kidneys increase the plasma bicarbonate

- Replacement of filtered bicarbonate with bicarbonate that is generated in the tubular cells
- Replacement of filtered phosphate with bicarbonate that is generated in the tubular cells
- By generation of 'new' bicarbonate from glutamine that is absorbed by the tubular cell

Define the base deficit.

The base deficit is the amount of acid or alkali required to restore 1 l of blood to a normal pH at a pCO_2 of 5.3 kPa and at 37°C. It is an indicator of the metabolic component to an acid–base disturbance. The normal range is -2 to $+2$ mmol/l.

ACUTE RENAL FAILURE

What is the definition of acute renal failure?

This is the inability of the kidney to excrete the nitrogenous and other waste products of metabolism and can develop over the course of a few hours or days. It is therefore a biochemical diagnosis

How are the causes basically classified?

The causes may be considered to be pre-renal, renal or post-renal.

What are the major 'renal' causes of acute renal failure?

- Acute tubular necrosis
- Glomerulonephritis
- Interstitial nephritis
- Bilateral cortical necrosis
- Reno-vascular: vasculitis, renal artery thrombosis
- Hepatorenal syndrome

What is acute tubular necrosis?

Acute tubular necrosis is renal failure resulting from injury to the tubular epithelial cells, and is the most important cause of acute renal failure. There are two types

- *Ischaemic injury:* following any cause of shock with resulting fall in the renal perfusion pressure and oxygenation

- *Nephrotoxic injury:* from drugs (aminoglycosides, paracetamol), toxins (heavy metals, organic solvents), or myoglobin (from rhabdomyolysis)

A

What are the major 'post-renal' causes?

- Acute obstruction from calculi
- Obstruction from tumours arising from the renal parenchyma or transitional epithelium of the pelvi-calyceal system
- Extrinsic compression from pelvic tumours
- Iatrogenic injury, e.g. inadvertent damage to the ureters during bowel surgery
- Prostatic obstruction
- Increased intra-abdominal pressure ($>30\,cmH_2O$)

Which part of the kidney is the most poorly perfused?

The renal medulla is more poorly perfused than the cortex. This ensures that the medullary interstitial concentration gradient formed by tubular counter current multiplication is preserved and maintained.

Which part of the nephron is the most susceptible to ischaemic injury, and why?

The cells of the thick ascending limb are the most susceptible to ischaemic injury for two important reasons

- The cells reside in the medulla, which has poorer oxygenation than the cortex
- The active Na^+-K^+ ATPase pumps at the cell membrane have a high oxygen demand

What are the basic steps in the pathogenesis of acute renal failure?

The basic steps in the pathogenesis are

- Initially, there is renal parenchymal ischaemia: as part of the compensatory response to a fall in the renal perfusion pressure, there is vasoconstriction of the efferent arteriole. Thus, by reducing the pre to post capillary resistance ratio, the capillary filtration pressure is preserved at the expense of reducing the blood supply to the tubules from the efferent arteriole and vasa recta. This leads to worsening cortical and medullary ischaemia

- Tubular cell ischaemia and necrosis leads to cells being shed into the tubular lumen, causing obstruction
- This promotes a 'back-leak' of tubular fluid into the interstitium, increasing the interstitial hydrostatic pressure
- This reduces tubular fluid reabsorption and worsens oliguria

Name some common drugs of surgical importance that may exacerbate or cause acute renal failure.

- *Paracetamol:* overdose is a known cause of acute tubular necrosis
- *Non-steroidal anti-inflammatory drugs:* can lead to renal failure by reducing the renal protective effects of prostaglandins during renal ischaemia
- *Aminoglycosides:* a potent cause of acute tubular necrosis
- *Penicillins:* can cause interstitial nephritis
- *Furosemide:* can lead to interstitial nephritis
- *Dextran 40:* a colloid used during fluid resuscitation

How is acute renal failure recognised?

Acute renal failure is a biochemical diagnosis:

- Oliguria (<400 ml of urine passed per day) may or may not be present
- Biochemical markers of reduced glomerular filtration rate: acutely elevated serum urea and creatinine
- Biochemical markers of diminished electrolyte homeostasis: hyponatraemia, hyperkalaemia, metabolic acidosis, hypocalcaemia
- Changes in the composition of the urine compared to the plasma: *see* table in 'Low urine output'

A

How may it be distinguished from chronic renal failure?

It may sometimes be difficult to distinguish from pre-existing chronic renal failure, but some clues may be gathered from different sources

- Previous blood results may suggest long-term renal suppression or deterioration
- There may be a progressive history of some of the signs and symptoms of chronic renal failure, such as skin pigmentation, chronic anaemia, pruritis or nocturia
- In chronic renal failure, ultrasound examination reveals small or scarred kidneys

What are the two most important life-threatening complications?

- *Acute pulmonary oedema:* due to fluid retention with over-hydration
- *Hyperkalaemia:* leading to metabolic acidosis and cardiac arrhythmias

Both may require urgent dialysis as part of the management.

What are the principles of management of established acute renal failure?

- Stop all nephrotoxic agents, and careful use of other drugs that undergo renal excretion
- Careful fluid balance: this is to ensure that the patient is not 'tipped' into acute pulmonary oedema. The daily input depends on the overall output. One regimen suggests that input and output should be equal, plus the addition of 500−1000 ml to account for insensible losses. Adequate fluid balance requires a daily fluid balance chart, daily examination and weighing of the patient
- Nutritional support: best performed by the enteral route, paying special attention to the protein input
- Management of complications mentioned above, including prophylaxis for GI bleeding with the use of H^+-antagonists

- Renal replacement therapies: dialysis or filtration
- Management of the underlying trigger, e.g. obstruction, sepsis, glomerulonephritis

What is the prognosis of acute renal failure?

Mortality of renal failure on its own is in the order of 5–10%. Depending on the cause, often there is good recovery of renal function within several weeks.

ACUTE RESPIRATORY DISTRESS SYNDROME (ARDS)

What is the definition of lung compliance?

Lung compliance is defined as the change in volume per unit change in pressure. The greater the compliance, the greater the volume increase achieved for a particular pressure change. The overall compliance of the lung is $0.2\,L/cmH_2O$.

What is lung surfactant composed of, and what purpose does it serve?

Surfactant is a phospholipid mixture (such as dipalmitoylphosphatidylcholine, other lipids and protein) produced by Type II pneumocytes. It has detergent-like properties in reducing the surface tension of the fluid lining the alveoli. Thus, according to Laplace's law, a smaller transpulmonary pressure is required to overcome the surface tension when inflating the alveolus.

What is the definition of ARDS?

ARDS is a syndrome of acute respiratory failure with the formation of a non-cardiogenic pulmonary oedema leading to reduced lung compliance and hypoxaemia which is refractory to oxygen therapy. The changes are seen as

- Diffuse pulmonary infiltrates seen on chest radiography
- Pulmonary wedge pressure of <16 mmHg, excluding pulmonary oedema due to elevated left atrial pressure
- PaO_2/FiO_2 ratio of <26.6 kPa (200 mmHg)

How does it relate to 'acute lung injury' and the 'systemic inflammatory response syndrome'?

Acute lung injury (ALI) comprises of a number of non-specific pathological changes in the lung in response to a specific insult. These changes are like that of ARDS, but of decreased severity in that the PaO_2/FiO_2 is <40 kPa (300 mmHg). Thus, ARDS can be considered to be at the extreme end of the spectrum of ALI. ARDS is the respiratory component to the systemic

▼

inflammatory response syndrome that is associated with multi-organ dysfunction.

What are the causes of ARDS?

The triggering factors can be organised into a number of groups

- Pulmonary insults:
  - Trauma
  - Pneumonia
  - Aspiration
  - Smoke inhalation
  - Fat embolism
- Multiple trauma
- Generalised sepsis
- Others: massive transfusion, disseminated intravascular coagulation (DIC), acute pancreatitis, cardio-pulmonary bypass

Discuss the process that leads to its effects on the lung.

The pathophysiological changes may be seen in the flow-diagram overleaf.

The histopathological changes are divided into a number of discrete phases that can take less than 24 h to establish:

- Inflammatory/exudative phase
  - Activated neutrophils and macrophages in the area release a number of mediators such as oxygen radicals, proteases, prostaglandins, tumour necrosis factor (TNF) and collagenases
  - There is local activation of the complement and coagulation cascades
  - Subsequent endothelial injury leads to increased capillary permeability and the formation of pulmonary oedema
  - Epithelial injury manifests as a decrease of Type-II pneumocytes, reducing surfactant production

▼

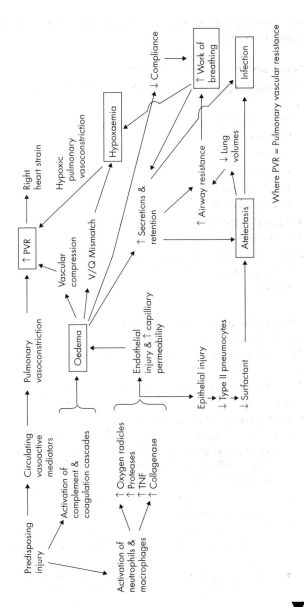

Where PVR = Pulmonary vascular resistance

- Proliferative phase: 5–10 days later
  - With a proliferation of Type-II pneumocytes
  - There is an increase in the local fibroblast population
- Progressive interstitial fibrosis

In consequence, there are a number of physiological changes in the lung

- Oedema and decreased lung volume leads to a fall in lung compliance, which increases the work of breathing
- Increased secretions and their retention give rise to local atelectasis and a reduction of the functional residual capacity
- Therefore, there is increased shunt and V/Q mismatch, leading to hypoxaemia and respiratory failure
- There is increased pulmonary vascular resistance caused by the oedema compressing the vessels, and by hypoxic pulmonary vasoconstriction occurring as a defense mechanism in order to improve the V/Q
- Atelectasis with pulmonary endothelial and epithelial injury predisposes to infection
- Pulmonary hypertension increases the work of the right heart, and can lead to right heart dysfunction
- Progressive interstitial fibrosis may persist even after the patient has recovered

What are the principles of management?

The principles of management lie in a number of supportive measures:

- Management of the initial predisposing insult
- Adequate nutritional support
- Mechanical ventilation to improve oxygenation and elimination of CO_2. High levels of positive end-expiratory pressure (PEEP) (10–20 cmH$_2$O) may be used to hold open the alveoli throughout the whole respiratory cycle, but at the cost of encouraging barotrauma to the lung
- Small tidal volumes have been shown to improve outcome. This leads to a permissive hypercarbia that is usually well tolerated

- Inverse ratio ventilation: normally the Inspiratory:Expiratory (I:E) ratio is 1:2, but the length of the inspiratory phase is increased to improve oxygenation of small obstructed airways
- Prone ventilation: patients are nursed in the prone position while receiving intermittent positive pressure ventilation (IPPV). This is thought to redistribute secretions and alter the V/Q, improving oxygenation
- Strict control of fluid resuscitation to prevent worsening pulmonary oedema
- Inhaled nitric oxide: this can be used in order to induce pulmonary vasodilatation (with no systemic vasodilatation), reducing pulmonary hypertension and improving the V/Q in the well–ventilated areas that receive it. However, the full benefits have yet to be proven
- Other unproven treatments: inhaled prostacyclin, steroids (may be of help in reducing the fibrotic process)

What is the prognosis?

The outcome generally is still poor, with 50–60% mortality. ARDS associated with sepsis has the poorest outcome, with a mortality of up to 90%.

What is the mechanism of action of nitric oxide?

Nitric oxide, ('endothelium–derived relaxing factor') is an activator of the cytoplasmic enzyme guanylyl cyclase. This increases the intracellular cyclic guanosine monophosphate (cGMP) levels, which stimulates a cGMP–dependent protein kinase. This activated protein kinase stimulate the phosphorylation of key proteins in a pathway that leads to a relaxation of vascular smooth muscle cells.

AGITATION AND SEDATION

Give some causes of acute confusion in the post–operative patient.

- Pain, anxiety and disorientation: all can commonly occur in ITU patients
- Sepsis: systemic infection, or localised to chest, urinary tract, wound etc
- Hypoglycaemia, or hyperglycaemia with ketoacidosis
- Respiratory failure, leading to hypoxaemia and/or hypercarbia: precipitating causes apart from chest infection include acute pulmonary oedema, pneumothorax, pulmonary embolism, and sputum retention/atelectasis
- Hypotension of any cause: e.g. bleeding, myocardial infarction, or arrhythmia leading to reduced cerebral perfusion
- Acute renal or hepatic failure
- Electrolyte disturbance: most commonly hypo or hypernatraemia
- Water imbalance: both dehydration and water overload
- Acute urinary retention – especially in the elderly
- Drugs: opiate analgesia, excess sedative drugs, anticholinergics

Which investigations should you perform?

A full history and examination must be carried out so that the most pertinent investigations are performed. These investigations include

- Arterial blood gas analysis: which determines the base excess and respiratory function
- Serum glucose
- Full blood count
- Serum electrolytes: sodium, potassium, calcium, phosphate, magnesium, lactate (strictly speaking, a metabolite), urea and creatinine

- Liver function tests
- Sepsis screen: blood cultures, wound swab, urine and sputum cultures
- Radiology: such as a chest radiograph
- ECG: for arrhythmias or myocardial infarction

What is the purpose of sedation in the critical care setting?

- Anxiolysis
- Analgesia
- Amnesia
- Hypnosis

Thus, there is a reduction in the level of consciousness, but with retention of verbal communication. There is much variability on which permutation of these effects individual agents produce.

Therefore, from a practical perspective in the intensive care setting, they are used to permit tolerance of endotracheal tubes, oral suction and other bed-side procedures.

How is the level of sedation determined?

There are a number of techniques in routine clinical use to determine the level of sedation attained. The most commonly employed of these is the Ramsay scoring system that describes six levels of sedation

- *Level 1:* The patient is anxious and agitated or restless or both
- *Level 2:* The patient is co-operative, orientated and tranquil
- *Level 3:* Responds to commands only
- *Level 4:* Asleep. Brisk response to glabellar tap or loud auditory stimulus
- *Level 5:* Asleep. Sluggish response to glabellar tap or loud auditory stimulus

A

- *Level 6:* Asleep. No response to glabellar tap or loud auditory stimulus

The ideally sedated patient attains levels 2–4.

Which classes of drugs may be used?

The most commonly used classes of drugs are

- *Benzodiazepines:* e.g. diazepam and midazolam
- *Intravenous (i.v.) anaesthetic agents:* such as propofol and ketamine
- *Inhalational anaesthetic:* nitrous oxide (70%)
- *Opiate analgesics:* morphine and the synthetic opioids pethidine and fentanyl are popular choices. They may be combined effectively with benzodiazepines
- *Trichloroethanol derivatives:* such as chloral hydrate
- *Butyrophenones:* e.g. haloperidol. As a group they are neurotransmitter-blocking drugs
- *Phenothiazines:* e.g. chlorpromazine. They also act on neurotransmitter receptors

Which of these are the most commonly used for sedation in critical care?

The most commonly used sedative drugs are propofol, benzodiazepines and the opioid analgesics.

What is the major physiological side effect of propofol?

The important side effect of propofol is hypotension on induction, and is caused by a fall in the systemic vascular resistance and/or myocardial depression. As with many of the other sedatives, it also leads to respiratory depression.

AIRWAY MANAGEMENT

A

How is the airway assessed clinically?

Assessment is based on the principle of: LOOK, LISTEN and FEEL.

- LOOK: For the presence of use of the accessory muscles of respiration, presence of obvious foreign bodies or facial/airway injury and the 'see-saw' pattern of obstructed respiration. Central cyanosis is a late sign
- LISTEN: For the presence of stridor, which indicates upper airways obstruction. Also grunting or gurgling
- FEEL: For chest wall movements and airflow at the nose

Note that in cases of trauma, the assessment has to be performed with cervical spine control.

What techniques of airway management do you know?

Broadly speaking, there are *simple* and *definitive* airway management techniques.

- Simple measures:
  - Rigid suction device to clear debris and secretions
  - Chin lift manoeuvre
  - Jaw thrust manoeuvre
  - Airway adjuncts: oropharnygeal and nasopharyngeal airways
- Definitive airway management:
  - Orotracheal intubation
  - Nasotracheal intubation
  - Surgical airway

How are the chin lift and jaw thrust manoeuvres performed?

Chin lift: The fingers of one hand are placed under the mandible in the mid-line, and then lifted upwards to bring the chin forward.

Jaw thrust: The angles of the lower jaw are grasped on both sides by the fingers, displacing the mandible forward.

▼

What do you know of the airway adjuncts?

The adjuncts are the

- *Oropharyngeal (Guedel) airway:* must not be inserted if there is a gag reflex present

- *Nasopharyngeal airway:* must not be inserted if a skull-base or cribriform plate fracture is suspected

What kinds of 'surgical' airway are there?

There are three types of surgical airway:

- Needle cricothyroidotomy with jet insufflation of oxygen
- Cricothyroidotomy
- Tracheostomy: which may be performed in the emergency or elective setting

What are the indications for a 'surgical' airway?

- Failed intubation, e.g. due to oedema
- Traumatic fracture of the larynx

In which anatomic location are the 'surgical' airways sited?

Both types of cricothyroidotomy are performed through the median cricothyroid ligament. This is the thickened anterior portion of the cricothyroid membrane that runs between the cricoid and thyroid cartilages.

A tracheostomy may be placed from the second to fifth tracheal rings, via a vertical slit. A tracheal flap of Bjork may also be fashioned, although less commonly used because of the risk of stenosis.

How is jet insufflation of oxygen performed, and what is the main precaution to be considered?

This is carried out by way of a needle passed into the airway through the median cricothyroid ligament. It is connected to a source of oxygen via a tracheal tube connector. The patient is well oxygenated but poorly ventilated, leading to progressive hypercarbia. In consequence, its use should be limited to a 45 min period which 'buys time' for a definitive airway to be established.

ANALGESIA

What class of analgesics are there?

The commonly-used agents may be categorised as

- Opiates
- Paracetamol (acetaminophen)
- NSAIDs
- Regional anaesthetic blockade, achieving analgesia

How may analgesics be administered?

The common routes of administration are

- Enteral: oral (including sublingual), rectal
- Parenteral:
  - i.v. infusion, including patient-controlled analgesia (PCA)
  - Intermittent intramuscular injection or regional infiltration of local anaesthetic
  - Intranasal: for opiates in the paediatric setting
  - Intrathecal route: epidural analgesia using bupivacaine
  - Inhalation: such as 70% nitrous oxide (a volatile anaesthetic)
  - Transcutaneous: such as fentanyl patches for chronic pain

Give some examples of the opiates in common use. Which are the synthetic and non-synthetic agents?

The commonly used opiates are

- *Non-synthetic:* morphine, codeine (10% of this is metabolised to morphine)
- *Semi-synthetic:* diamorphine, dihydrocodeine
- *Synthetic:* pethidine, fentanyl

Which receptor do opiate analgesics act on?

The majority of the effects of the opiates are carried out through the μ-receptor. They may also have some action through the other two types of opiate receptors, κ and δ.

A

What are the systemic effects of the opiates?

The effects of the opiates are

- *Analgesia:* they are good for moderate to severe pain of any cause and modality. Less effective for neuropathic pain, such as phantom limb pain, or allodynia (pain from a non-painful stimulus)

- *Respiratory depression:* with blunting of the ventilatory response to rising pCO_2. Also causes suppression of the cough reflex, both of which encourage sputum retention, atelectasis and pneumonia in the critically ill

- *Sedation:* with a reduction in the level of consciousness with higher doses, so beware in those with head injuries

- *Nausea and vomiting:* following stimulation of the chemoreceptor trigger zone in the area postrema

- *Reduced GI motility:* which leads to constipation

- *Euphoria*

- *Dependence and tolerance:* there is a progressively reduced effect from the same dose of drug

- *Histamine release from mast cells:* producing pruritis and reduced systemic vascular resistance

Why is morphine not advocated for use in abdominal pain of biliary origin?

Morphine increases the tone of the sphincter of Oddi (as well other sphincteric muscles), while stimulating contraction of the gallbladder. Therefore, it can exacerbate biliary pain.

Which drug is given for opiate overdose? What is the mechanism of action?

Naloxone may be used to reverse the effects of opioids. This is a short-acting μ-receptor antagonist. Note that because of its short duration of action, the effects of the opioids may return after an initial reversal.

A

What are the therapeutic effects of paracetamol (acetaminophen)?

This is an analgesic and anti-pyretic with minimal anti-inflammatory properties.

By what mechanism does overdose cause liver injury?

The cause of liver injury lies with the metabolism of para-cetamol. Normally it is conjugated in the liver, with the production of a small amount of the toxic metabolite N-acetyl-benzoquinoneimine. Binding to hepatic glutathione renders this metabolite harmless. With overdose, glutathione is depleted, leading to hepatocyte injury. Acetylcycteine, the drug used to treat overdose, is a glutathione precursor.

How do the non-steroidal anti-inflammatory drugs (NSAIDs) work?

These agents act to reduce prostaglandin formation by the inhibition of the enzyme cyclo-oxygenase which acts on arachidonic acid. This leads to a modification of the inflammatory reaction and its effects on the stimulating nociception.

What are NSAIDs systemic side effects?

The systemic side-effects of these agents include

- *Gastrointestinal:* dyspepsia, gastritis and peptic ulceration. There is direct stimulation of acid secretion by the gastric parietal cells, with reduced bicarbonate and mucus production

- *Renal:* may precipitate acute renal failure, especially in those with pre-existing renal suppression, dehydration or hypotension. Also leads to salt and water retention

- *Coagulopathy:* inhibition of platelet thromboxane A2 production leads to their reduced ability to aggregate and form the primary platelet plug. This is a permanent effect, and is reversed only when new platelets are formed

- *Bronchospasm:* the inhibition of cyclo-oxygenase leads to arachidonic acid being metabolised down the pathway of leukotriene formation, which induce brochospasm

▼

How is renal injury precipitated?

There is inhibition of compensatory PGI2 and PGE2 formation that occurs during situations of reduced renal perfusion. These prostaglandins normally promote vasodilatation during such situations, offsetting the development of acute tubular necrosis.

What local anaesthetic techniques are available for pain relief?

The local anaesthetic techniques available are

- *Local nerve blocks:* such as the 3 in 1 block of the lateral cutaneous, femoral and obturator nerves that can be used for fractured neck of femur. Also intercostal block following chest injury or thoracotomy

- *Caudal block:* strictly speaking a form of epidural anaesthesia particularly useful for paediatric practise

- *Epidural and spinal block:* the former is more popular because of its longer duration of action and reduced systemic adverse effects

When is epidural analgesia commonly employed?

Epidural analgesia is commonly used in the post-operative setting, being especially useful in situations where pain may compromise respiratory function, e.g. thoracic or upper abdominal surgery.

Why is epidural analgesia's use limited in the critical care setting?

- The patient may be septic or have a local infection: both of which contraindicate the use of an epidural

- Epidurals must not be inserted in the presence of a coagulopathy

- The patient may not be able to consent owing to lack of consciousness

- The patient may be hypovolaemic, leading to decompensated hypotension in those with an epidural

A

What are the potential systemic effects of this form of analgesia?

Some of the systemic effects of epidurals include

- *Hypotension:* due to block of the sympathetic outflow causing peripheral vasodilatation
- Reduced cardiac output may occur due to a reduction in the venous return
- Attenuation of the surgical stress response
- Reduction of the functional residual capacity
- Reduction of post-operative deep venous thrombosis: due to a number of causes including the concomitant use of i.v. fluids used to support the arterial pressure

AORTIC DISSECTION

How are aortic dissections classified?

Aortic dissections may be classified according to the Stanford or DeBakey systems

- Stanford
  - *Type A:* dissection involves the ascending aorta only
  - *Type B:* involves the descending aorta with or without the ascending aorta
- DeBakey
  - *Type I:* involves the ascending aorta, arch and descending aorta
  - *Type II:* confined to the ascending aorta
  - *Type III:* confined to the descending aorta, beyond the origin of the subclavian artery

What are the pathological hallmarks of dissection?

The recognised findings on microscopy are

- *Myxoid degeneration:* loss of elastic fibres and replacement of the musculo-elastic tissue with a proteoglycan–rich matrix
- *Cystic medial necrosis:* may be associated with injury or occlusion of the vasa vasorum

In which plane of cleavage does the dissection propagate down the aorta?

Although initially commencing as an intimal tear, the dissection propagates along the plane that runs between the inner 2/3 and outer 1/3 of the media.

Which conditions predispose to aortic dissection?

The predisposing factors are

- Inherited defects:
  - *Marfan's syndrome:* there is defective cross-linking of collagen
  - *Ehlers-Danlos syndrome:* defective procollagen formation

- *Pseudoxanthoma elasticum:* fragmentation of elastic fibres in the media
- Hypertension: leading to increased shearing forces across the intima
- Pregnancy: associated with microscopic changes in the media
- Bicuspid aortic valve
- Traumatic injury to the aorta
- Iatrogenic: cardiac catheterisation, aortic cannulation at cardiac surgery, aortic valve replacement

What are the effects of dissection?

Dissection can lead to a number of outcomes

- Propagation to the abdominal aorta, leading to gut ischaemia if the mesenteric vessels are involved, or renal failure if the renal vessels are involved
- If the intercostal and lumbar vessels are occluded, then it can lead to spinal cord ischaemia, due to loss of the supply from the arteria radicularis magna
- Propagation along the carotid arteries, leading to stroke
- Involvement of the coronary ostia and coronary arteries: leading to angina and myocardial infarction
- Involvement of the aortic valve ring, with the development of acute aortic regurgitation
- Rupture into the pericardium, producing cardiac tamponade
- Rupture into the pleura, producing a haemothorax
- Compression of surrounding structures: such as the trachea, oesophagus or superior vena cava
- The dissection may re-enter the lumen through another intimal tear, producing a double-barreled aorta

What may the physical examination show?

Some findings on physical examination

- The patient may exhibit signs of cardiogenic or hypovolaemic shock

- New diastolic murmur of aortic regurgitation
- Signs of cardiac tamponade: muffled heart sounds, increased venous pressure, reduced arterial pressure and pulsus paradoxus
- Asymmetric pulses and blood pressures
- Neurological signs: stroke or spinal cord involvement

Which investigations may be employed in making the diagnosis?

Note that the purpose of investigation is to

- Make the correct diagnosis from the list of differentials
- Assess the extent of the dissection to help plan management
- Discover the presence of complications: such as myocardial infarction
- Discover the presence of any other co-morbidities that can complicate management

There are a number of investigations that help in establishing the diagnosis and assess the severity.

- *ECG:* will establish the presence of myocardial infarction, and exclude cardiac differential diagnoses

- *Chest radiograph:* abnormal in 80% of cases; may show a widened mediastinum, displacement of the aortic knuckle, depression of the left main bronchus, or a haemothorax.

- *Angiography:* the gold standard that allows visualisation of ventricular and valve function, and permits assessment of coronary anatomy. However, it is invasive, and the contrast dye may worsen renal dysfunction

- *CT/MRI scanning:* has a sensitivity and specificity of 85 and >90% respectively. Permits spiral CT imaging. Does not provide information on cardiac function

- *Trans-oesophageal echocardiography:* sensitivity and specificity of >95%. Has the advantage that it can used at the bedside, and can assess cardiac function and valve involvement

How is aortic dissection managed?

The principles of management include

- Adequate resuscitation with fluids to maintain the cardiac index and renal function. Following bladder catheterisation, a urine output of 30–40 ml/h must be maintained

- The fluids are given through wide-bore i.v. cannulae, from which samples can be taken for baseline investigations and a 10-unit cross match of blood

- A central-line should be inserted to help monitor the filling pressures

- The velocity of the ejection fraction and arterial pressure should be controlled with an infusion of labetalol. Sodium nitroprusside has also been used, but this can cause a reflex tachycardia and increases the ejection velocity. This increases the shearing forces on the intima, propagating the dissection

- The patient should be transferred to a cardiothoracic unit when stable

- Surgery involves replacement of the diseased segment of the aorta with a prosthetic graft and re-implantation of the coronary arteries if the aortic root is involved

- Aortic root involvement also requires valve replacement or re-suspension

- If the arch is involved, deep hypothermic circulatory arrest is required during repair to preserve cerebral function

- For type B dissections, conservative management is advocated – surgery confers no added benefit

- In some instances, the dissection may be stented

ATELECTASIS

What is the definition of atelectasis?

Atelectasis is defined as an absence of gas from all or part of the lung.

What causes atelectasis and what is the pathophysiology?

The aetiology includes

- Bronchial obstruction: by sputum, foreign body, tumour
- Alveolar hypoventilation: leading to progressive absorption of gas and subsequent collapse of the parenchyma
- Parenchymal compression by pleural effusion or pulmonary oedema
- Inadvertent endobronchial intubation: with collapse of the unventilated lung parenchyma

In the case of airways obstruction, there is distal gas trapping. This trapped gas is absorbed since it has a higher partial pressure than that of the mixed venous blood. This leads to progressive collapse of the lung beyond the obstruction. The physiological consequence is

- V/Q mismatch and hypoxaemia
- Reduction of lung compliance (as can be seen from the lung's compliance curve), with a consequent increase in the work of breathing
- Predisposition to infection due to retention of secretions

Why does a high-inspired concentration of oxygen lead to atelectasis?

The reason lies in the higher solubility and faster absorption of oxygen as compared with nitrogen. When inspiring air, the slowly absorbed nitrogen 'splints' the airways open as oxygen is being absorbed. At a high FiO_2, this nitrogen 'splint' is reduced or absent, so that when the oxygen is absorbed, the lung unit collapses. This is also called 'absorption' atelectasis.

A

What are the risk factors for post-operative atelectasis?

- Upper abdominal and thoracic surgery: reduced lung expansion from pain and diaphragmatic splinting leads to retention of secretions and distal airways collapse
- Body mass index of >27
- Smoking
- Age over 60
- COPD

What are the principles of post-operative atelectasis management?

- *Preoperative anticipation:* breathing exercises before the operation may be used to improve expansion
- *Intra-operative management:*
  - Humidification which improves mucociliary function
  - Adequate tidal volumes to ensure good expansion
  - Avoid unnecessarily high FiO_2 to prevent "absorption atelectasis"
- *Post-operative measures:*
  - Position the patient upright
  - Adequate analgesia to encourage good tidal volumes
  - Mobilise early
  - Breathing exercises
  - CPAP
  - Airway suction to clear secretions

Note that deep-breathing exercises aid lung expansion. As the lung expands, the compliance improves (as seen from the compliance curve) and, through the process of radial traction, the airflow resistance falls. Both these factors contribute to a reduction in the work of breathing.

What is continuous positive airway pressure (CPAP) ventilation, and what are its physiological effects on the respiratory system?

CPAP is an oxygen delivery system that relies on a closed circuit to provide positive airways pressure throughout all phases of spontaneous ventilation. The circuit can be attached to a tracheal tube or to a tight fitting mask, which means that it may be used on the ward under supervision. Some of the physiological methods by which it improves alveolar ventilation are

- Recruitment of collapsed alveoli, and prevention of their collapse on expiration
- Increase in the functional residual capacity (FRC): in the elderly and critically ill, collapse of the airways occurs close to the volume of the FRC. By increasing the FRC, atelectasis can be avoided or overcome
- Increased lung compliance, reducing the work of breathing
- Consequently the V/Q ratio increases, improving oxygenation

What are the disadvantages of CPAP ventilation?

- The tight fitting mask is uncomfortable and may be poorly tolerated
- Causes gastric dilatation due to swallowed air
- Barotrauma to the alveoli due to high pressures (more common in neonates)

BLOOD PRESSURE MONITORING

Define the blood pressure.
Blood pressure is defined as the product of the cardiac output and the systemic vascular resistance. The cardiac output is the product of the heart rate and stroke volume.

In which ways can blood pressure be measured?
Blood pressure can be measured non-invasively with a sphygmomanometer, or invasively by direct cannulation of a peripheral artery. This latter method gives a continuous waveform trace after attachment to an electronic pressure transducer.

Draw the blood pressure waveform.

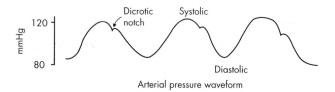

Arterial pressure waveform

The 'dicrotic notch' is a momentary rise in the arterial pressure trace following closure of the aortic valve.

How is the mean blood pressure calculated?
The area beneath the arterial pressure wave tracing represents the mean arterial pressure. For the purposes of simplicity, it may be calculated by the formula

Pd + (Ps − Pd)/3

where Pd = diastolic pressure and Ps = systolic pressure.

What is Allen's test, and how is it performed?
Allen's test is a test of the competence of the collateral circulation of the hand – and may be used practically to determine

if the ulnar artery supply to the hand is able to cope in the face of an absent radial artery, e.g. when considering the use of the radial artery as a vascular conduit for bypass surgery.

The examiner occludes the blood flow to the hand while the patient drains the hand of blood by repeatedly opening and closing the fist. The hand is then held open while the ulnar flow is released. The test is considered positive if the hand is still blanched after 15 s, suggesting that the ulnar artery alone is not able to sufficiently supply the hand.

What are the complications of arterial lines, and what are the contra-indications to their insertion?

The complications include

- Most commonly:
  - Haematoma formation
  - Digital ischaemia due to vascular injury or accidental injection of drugs
- Less commonly:
  - Infection
  - Pseudoaneurysm formation
  - Arteriovenous fistula formation
  - Exsanguination from a disconnected line

It is contra-indicated in those with digital vasculitis, and in those patients who are going to have the artery of that side harvested as a conduit for bypass surgery.

What is meant by the term '*swing in the arterial line*' during continuous measurements, and what is its significance?

This term refers to a variation of the amplitude in the arterial tracing with the respiratory cycle. It is an indicator that the patient is underfilled and requires more fluid resuscitation.

How does the arterial pressure at the radial artery compare to that at the aortic root, what accounts for this difference?

Both the pressure values and waveform change at different levels of the circulation. In the radial artery, the systolic pressure is about 10 mmHg higher and the diastolic pressure about 10 mmHg lower than in the aortic root. Consequently, although the pulse pressure is higher in the radial artery, the mean arterial pressure is about 5 mmHg lower than in the aortic root.

These differences are, in part, due to changes in wall stiffness along the arterial tree, and its consequent effects on the transmission of the pulse wave along the vessel.

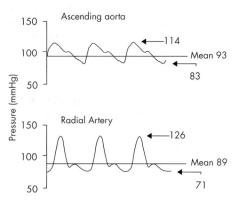

Pressure waves at different sites in the arterial tree. With transmission of the pressure wave into the distal aorta and large arteries, the systolic pressure increases and the diastolic pressure decreases, with a resultant heightening of the pulse pressure. However, the mean arterial pressure declines steadily.

Adapted from "Circulatory Physiology"
3rd edition by Smith & Kampire p 93
Published by Williams & Wilkins
ISBN 0683077759

How does the arterial pressure waveform differ with diseases of the aortic valve?

- *Aortic stenosis:* Anacrotic pulse – slow to rise and of low amplitude

- *Aortic incompetence:* Waterhammer pulse – rapid rise and decline, attaining high amplitude

- *Mixed aortic valve disease:* Pulsus bisferiens – a large amplitude pulse with a 'double peak', often felt as a double pulse at the brachial artery

What is pulsus paradoxus?

Pulsus paradoxus is an exaggerated (>10 mmHg) reduction of the arterial pressure brought on by inspiration, and may be seen in cardiac tamponade. The normal increase in the venous return brought on by inspiration coupled with a tight pericardial space leads to a reduction of the left ventricular end diastolic volume, and hence, stroke volume.

What is pulsus alterans?

Pulsus alterans is a random variation in the amplitude of the arterial pressure tracing with each cardiac cycle, and is seen with left ventricular failure.

BLOOD PRODUCTS

What blood products do you know of other than red cells?

The other major blood products are
- Plasma-derived
  - Fresh frozen plasma (FFP)
  - Human albumin solution
  - Immunoglobulins
  - Individual factor concentrates, e.g. factors VII, VIII, IX, X, prothrombin complex, antithrombin III
  - Cryoprecipitate

Note that FFP may be fractionated into the products listed below it.
- Platelet concentrates

How are platelets stored once collected?

Platelets do not function at low temperatures, so that once collected, they are stored at room temperature of 20–24°C on a special agitator.

What is the shelf life of platelets?

This is 5–7 days if sealed in special packaging that permits atmospheric oxygenation.

How many platelets are obtained from each donation?

Each platelet donation contains 55×10^9 platelets. When pooled together to form an adult dose, about 240×10^9 platelets can be obtained.

Give some indications for a platelet transfusion.

These are basically
- Any cause of thrombocytopenia, when the count falls below $50 \times 10^9/l$
- Note that the above includes disseminated intravascular coagulation

- Post cardiopulmonary bypass: It is known that this has a direct detrimental effect on platelet function. Also, patients coming off bypass may still have a low body temperature, which reduces platelet function. They may also have taken aspirin up to the time of surgery. Platelets may in these instances be required to control bleeding even though the platelet count may not be that low

What are the problems associated with platelet transfusion?

- *Risk of infection:* as for a transfusion of packed red cells

- *Rhesus sensitisation:* Rh negative females under the age of 45 should receive Rh-D negative platelets

- *Alloimmunisation:* this is due to development of antibodies to HLA class I antigens. It can lead to a febrile transfusion reaction and 'refractoriness' to therapy, when the platelet count rises less than expected following a transfusion

What are the two main components of FFP?

The two main components are cryoprecipitate and cryosupernatant. Taken together, they are a rich source of all of the clotting factors, von Willebrand factor, fibrinogen, and other plasma proteins.

How is FFP stored and what is the shelf life?

FFP is stored at $-30°C$ for up to 12 months. Once thawed, it should be transfused immediately to prevent the loss of the labile factors V and VIII.

What is the dose of FFP?

The dose of FFP is weight-dependent, and a typical starting dose is 10–15 ml/kg.

Give some indications for its (FFP) use.

- Reversal of warfarin effect
- Help control intra-operative/post-operative bleeding, e.g. after cardiac surgery
- Following massive blood transfusion
- Disseminated intravascular coagulation
- Those with antithrombin III deficiency and resistance to heparinisation

What components is cryoprecipitate particularly rich in?

Cryoprecipitate is a rich source of fibrinogen, fibronectin, factors VIII, XIII (fibrin-stabilising factor), and von Willebrand factor.

What is the management of warfarin overdose?

The management of warfarin overdose depends on the severity of the blood loss and the international normalised ratio (INR).

- If the INR is >4.5 with no haemorrhage, the warfarin can be omitted for 1–2 days followed by a review
- If haemorrhage is not severe, warfarin may again be omitted, and if indicated clinically, reversed with a slow i.v. infusion of vitamin K, 0.5–2.0 mg
- In the face of severe haemorrhage, 5 mg of vitamin K is given by slow i.v. infusion together with prothrombin complex concentrate (PCC), containing factors II, IX and X with factor VII. Alternatively, FFP can be given, but may be less effective than PCC
- These guidelines are based on the advice of the 'Handbook of Transfusion Medicine' published by Her Majesty's Stationery Office (HMSO)

What types of human albumin are available?

Human albumin solution is available as either a 4.5% or 20% solution. The latter is also known as 'salt-poor albumin' since it contains less sodium.

What is the use of this blood product?

Some uses for human albumin

- Management of ascites in portal hypertension
- Oedema due to other causes of hypoalbuminaemia such as the nephrotic syndrome
- As a plasma expander in hypovolaemic shock: there is no evident superiority over other colloids or crystalloids in this situation

BLOOD TRANSFUSION

What is the purpose of a blood transfusion?

To restore the circulating volume in order to improve tissue perfusion and to maintain an adequate blood oxygen carrying capacity.

What is the volume of a unit of packed red cells?

280 ± 60 ml.

At what temperature is the blood stored?

2–6°C.

What is the shelf life of blood?

35 days, at the correct storage temperature.

What are the additive solutions and what is their purpose?

The most common additive solutions are

- CAPD: Citrate, Adenine, Phosphate, and Dextrose
- SAMG: Saline, Adenine, Mannitol, and Glucose

The additive solutions are used to re-suspend the packed cells after the plasma has been removed, and they maintain the cells in a good condition during storage.

What is the expected increase in the haemoglobin concentration [Hb] following a transfusion of packed red cells?

A 4 ml/kg dose of packed cells raises the [Hb] by 1 g/dl.

What is the estimated blood volume in an adult and a child?

The estimated blood volume in an adult is 70 ml/kg, in a child is 80 ml/kg.

For which infections is donated blood screened?

- Hepatitis B
- Hepatitis C
- HIV 1 and 2
- Syphilis

In special circumstances, e.g. for use in the immuno-compromised, CMV is screened.

How may the complications of blood transfusion be classified?

- Complications of massive transfusion
- Complications of repeated transfusion
- Infective complications
- Immune reactions

Define "*massive transfusion*" and what are the potential problems?

A *massive transfusion* is defined as a transfusion equaling the patients' blood volume within 24 h. The potential problems are

- *Volume overload* – can lead to acute pulmonary oedema in the susceptible

- *Thrombocytopenia:* following storage there is a reduction of functioning platelets, so that there is a dilutional thrombocytopenia following a large transfusion

- *Coagulation factor deficiency* – leading to a coagulopathy. May require blood products such as FFP for reversal

- Ineffective tissue oxygenation due to reduced of 2,3 bisphosphoglycerate, which does not store well

- *Hypothermia*

- *Hypocalcaemia:* Due to chelation by the citrate in the additive solution. May compound the coagulation defect

- *Hyperkalaemia:* Due to progressive potassium leakage from the stored red cells

Which coagulation factors are most affected by storage?

The most labile of the coagulation factors are V and VIII. The reduction of factor VIII may be offset by the metabolic response to stress, which stimulates factor VIII production.

What infective complications may be seen following transfusion?

- Hepatitis B and C
- HIV
- Syphilis
- *Yersinia enterocolitica:* Gram negative organism often implicated in red cell transfusions
- Gram positive infections, especially staphylococcal following contamination
- Infections associated with endemic areas: Malaria, Chaga's disease

What would make you suspect that a unit of blood has bacterial contamination?

- Presence of clots in the bag
- High degree of haemolysed red cells

Which immune reactions may occur following transfusion?

Immune reactions seen are

- *Febrile reaction:* Occurs within an hour of commencement as a reaction to white cell antigens in the donated blood

- *Acute haemolytic reaction* following ABO-incompatibility. This is usually due to a clerical error

- *Delayed haemolytic reaction:* The patient is immunised to foreign red cell antigens due to previous exposure. Can lead to jaundice and haemolysis days later

- *Post transfusion purpuric reaction:* Occurs 7–10 days following transfusion due to reaction to platelet PIAI antigens

- *Graft vs. Host disease:* A rare but almost-uniformly fatal reaction. Immunocompetent donor lymphocytes mediate an immune reaction to the recipient

- *Anaphylactic reaction*

How is the risk of Graft vs. Host disease reduced?

This is prevented by irradiation of the sample, and not through the use of leukocyte-depleted blood. Leukocyte depletion reduces the risk of CMV transmission.

What are the signs and symptoms of an immediate haemolytic transfusion reaction?

- Pyrexia and rigors
- Headache
- Abdominal and loin pain
- Facial flushing
- Hypotension, progressing to acute renal failure, disseminated intravascular coagulation (DIC) and acute lung injury

How is an immediate haemolytic transfusion reaction managed, and which investigations would you perform?

- Stop the transfusion immediately
- Commence i.v. fluid resuscitation, ensuring that the urine output is greater than 30–40 ml/h
- Repeat grouping on the pre- and post-transfusion recipient sample
- Repeat the cross match
- Perform a direct anti-globulin (Coomb's test) on the recipient post-transfusion sample
- Look for the presence of DIC – increased fibrin-degradation products, coagulopathy
- Check for evidence of the response to intravascular haemolysis – increased bilirubin, reduced circulating

haptoglobins, haemoglobinaemia, and haemoglobinuria.
Monitor this for 24 h

- Send samples for blood culture in case this was, in fact,
  a septic episode in response to contaminated blood

What is a direct Coomb's test?

Coomb's test, also known as a direct antiglobulin test, is used
for the detection of antibody or complement on the surface
of red cells that have developed *in vivo*. The indirect Coomb's
test detects red cell binding that has developed
in vitro. The direct test can be used in the detection of cases of

- Haemolytic transfusion reactions
- Haemolytic disease of the newborn
- Autoimmune haemolytic anaemias

BRAINSTEM DEATH AND ORGAN DONATION

Which organs may be donated?

- Kidneys
- Heart
- Lungs
- Liver
- Pancreas
- Small bowel
- Corneas
- Skin
- Bone and tendon

What are the general criteria that must be met prior to donation?

- The diagnosis of brainstem death must be established
- The donor is maintained on a ventilator in the absence of untreated sepsis
- There must not be a history of malignancy. Primary brain tumours are exempt because of the confined nature of the disease
- The donor must be HIV and hepatitis B negative
- Those from high-risk groups, such as i.v. drug abusers are excluded

There is some variation on these requirements depending on the organ to be donated, such as no history of myocardial infarction for heart donors, and no history of alcohol abuse among liver donors. Note that those with diabetes mellitus, smokers and those with hepatitis C are not immediately excluded.

Which law governs organ donation in the UK?

In the UK, donation of human organs is managed under the control of the Human Tissue Act of 1961.

Why is attention to fluid balance particularly important when optimising the physiology of the organ donor?

Those with brainstem death develop rapidly diabetes insipidus following loss of posterior pituitary function. This leads to free water loss, manifesting as a large urine output (>4 ml/kg/h), together with rising plasma osmolality and hypernatraemia. It may be corrected temporarily with i.v. dextrose. In severe cases, management requires an infusion of arginine vasopressin to control urine output.

What other physiological changes may occur with brainstem death?

- *Development of hypothermia:* following the loss of temperature regulation at the hypothalamic level. This is exacerbated by reduced muscular and metabolic activity together with peripheral vasodilatation. It is managed with the use of surface heating and warmed i.v. fluids. Note that hypothermia needs to be corrected before a diagnosis of brainstem death can be made correctly

- *Coagulopathy* may result from hypothermia

- *Initial hypertension:* due to an immediate increase in sympathetic activity. This can lead to cardiovascular instability with arrhythmia formation

- *Hypotension* soon follows due to the loss of sympathetic peripheral vascular tone. This may require inotropic support of the mean arterial pressure and organ perfusion

- *Endocrine changes:* following loss of anterior pituitary function. The most important consequence is loss of thyroid hormone production, leading to further arrhythmias. Triiodo-thyronine infusions have been used to help stabilise the patient in these situations

Under which circumstances is it appropriate to perform an examination to confirm brainstem death?

Clinical evaluation of the patient for the diagnosis of brainstem death must be justified, and so some preconditions must be met

▼

- The patient must be in a deep coma and reliant entirely on mechanical ventilation due to complete absence of spontaneous ventilation ('apnoeic coma')
- There should be irreversible brain damage that is compatible with a diagnosis of brainstem death

Those with the following, potentially reversible causes of coma should be identified and excluded

- Drug and alcohol intoxication
- Endocrine disturbances: such as hypothyroidism, uraemic or hepatic encephalopathy
- Metabolic disturbances: such as hypoglycaemia, or sodium imbalance
- Hypothermia with a core temperature of <35°C

What are the criteria for clinical confirmation of brainstem death?

The tests involve both an evaluation of the brainstem reflexes and the respiratory drive.

- Lack of respiratory drive following progressive hypercarbia: The subject is pre-oxygenated with 100% oxygen, and then disconnected from the ventilator for 10 min while the $PaCO_2$ is permitted to rise. Normally, respiration is stimulated above a $PaCO_2$ of 6.5 kPa.
- No brainstem function
  - Absent pupillary light reflex
  - Absent corneal reflex
  - Absent cranial nerve motor function
  - Absent gag and cough reflex following pharyngeal and bronchial stimulation with a catheter
  - Absent vestibulo-ocular test following a cold caloric test

The test should be repeated after an unspecified length of time for full confirmation.

Who may legally perform these tests?

The test must be performed by two clinicians who work in relevant areas of expertise, such as intensive care, anaesthesia, neurology or neurosurgery. One of them should be a consultant, and the other must have been registered with the General Medical Council for at least five years. They should not be part of the transplant team.

Under which clinical circumstances can confirmation prove difficult?

- Chronic obstructive pulmonary disease
- Eye injuries or pre-existing eye disease
- Brain-stem encephalitis

BRONCHIECTASIS

What do you understand by the term 'bronchiectasis'?

This is a localised or generalised irreversible dilatation of the bronchi arising as a result of a chronic necrotising infection. It is classed as one of the obstructive airways diseases.

What are the types of bronchiectasis?

There are three overlapping pathologic forms of bronchiectasis

- *Follicular:* characterised by the loss of bronchial elastic tissue and multiple lymphoid follicles

- *Atelectatic:* a localised dilatation of the airways, associated with parenchymal collapse due to proximal airways obstruction

- *Saccular:* which exhibits patchy dilatation of the airways. In this situation, there is a loss of the normal bronchial subdivisions

What is the aetiology of bronchiectasis?

A number of disease processes lead to bronchiectasis, but the basic pathogenesis involves cycles of acute and chronic inflammation accompanied by tissue damage and repair. Some of the more common causes are

- *Bronchial obstruction:* tumours, inhaled foreign body, extrinsic compression from lymphadenopathy

- *Infective processes:* bacterial and viral pneumonias, e.g. TB, measles, whooping cough, adenovirus

- *Mucociliary clearance defects:* Kartagener's and Young's syndromes, cystic fibrosis

- Primary and secondary immune deficiency states

Which bacteria may colonise the airways in those with bronchiectasis?

Bacterial colonisation often involve

- *Haemophilus influenzae*

- *Streptococcus pneumoniae*

- *Pseudomonas aeruginosa:* in the chronically afflicted

What complications can occur in the untreated patient with bronchiectasis?

- In the short term:
  - Haemoptysis – which may be severe
  - Recurrent chest infections, lung abscess, empyema
  - Metastatic infection, e.g. cerebral abscess
- Long term:
  - Respiratory failure due to chronic airway obstruction
  - Cor pulmonale secondary to pulmonary hypertension
  - Secondary amyloidosis with protein A deposition

How is bronchiectasis managed?

The principles of management involve

- Management of reversible airway obstruction with bronchodilators and inhaled steroids
- Physiotherapy to encourage expectoration of retained secretions. Patients may also be trained to perform postural drainage techniques
- Control of infection with antibiotics. This depends on the organism isolated, but popular choices are cefaclor, ciprofloxacin or amoxycillin. Prophylactic antibiotics have also been used
- Management of the underlying causes, e.g. airways obstruction, cystic fibrosis
- Surgical intervention has also been used, such as lobectomy for localised disease. In many instances, the disease is too diffuse to perform this. Transplantation has also been used for complicated bronchiectasis

BURNS

B

How common are burn injuries in the UK?

In the UK burns account for 10,000 hospital admissions and 600 deaths per annum.

What types of burns are there?

Burns may be

- Thermal: due to extreme heat or cold
- Electrical
- Chemical burns due to caustic substances

What criteria may be used for the assessment of thermal burns?

Burns are assessed by their extent on the body and their depth of skin penetration.

- *Extent:* described in terms of the percentage (%) body surface area covered. As a rule of thumb, the area covered by the patients' palm is equivalent to 1%. Also by the 'rule of nines': anterior and posterior trunk = 18%, head and arms = 9%, legs = 18% and genitalia = 1%
- *Depth:* may be superficial, partial or full-thickness: the clinical determinants of the depth are
  - Presence of erythema: seen in superficial burns
  - Blisters
  - Texture: leathery skin seen with full thickness burns
  - Sensation: burns are painful in areas where there is no full thickness penetration

Why are burns patients susceptible to respiratory complications?

- There may be a thermal injury to the nose or oropharynx with upper airway oedema
- Smoke inhalation can lead to hypoxia with pulmonary oedema from ARDS

▼

- Inhalation of carbon monoxide
- Inhalation of other toxic gases such as cyanide, or the oxides of sulphur and nitrogen
- Circumferential burns of the chest may restrict respiration
- Aggressive fluid resuscitation may produce pulmonary oedema
- A superadded chest infection may complicate pulmonary oedema

Why is carbon monoxide toxic?

- Its affinity for haemoglobin (forming carboxyhaemoglobin) is about 250 times greater than that of oxygen
- Consequently, the oxygen dissociation curve is shifted to the *left*, with poorer oxygenation of the tissues
- It also binds to some of the respiratory chain enzymes, such as cytochrome oxidase. Therefore, affecting oxygen utilisation at the cellular level

When would you become suspicious of an impeding respiratory problem?

- Fire in a confined space
- Soot at the mouth or in the sputum
- Burns on the face, singeing of the eyebrows
- Hoarse voice
- Serum carboxyhaemoglobin of >10%

Why are burns patients susceptible to renal failure?

- Hypovolaemia from plasma loss reduces the renal perfusion with the development of acute tubular necrosis
- Circulating myoglobin produces rhabdomyolysis, resulting in tubular injury and acute tubular necrosis
- Renal failure may occur as a complication of sepsis and the systemic inflammatory response

What are the other systemic complications of severe burns?

Aside from respiratory and renal failure, the other systemic complications are

- 'Burns shock': hypovolaemic shock due to plasma loss following loss of skin cover. Leads to hypotension, tachycardia, increased systemic vascular resistance and a fall in the cardiac output
- Electrolyte disturbances: Hypo or hypernatraemia, hyperkalaemia, hypocalcaemia
- Hypothermia following loss of skin cover – convection heaters may be used
- Systemic inflammatory response syndrome (SIRS) that can lead to multi-organ dysfunction and high mortality
- Generalised sepsis from organisms that include Clostridia. The features indicating sepsis may be indistinguishable from other causes of SIRS
- Gastric ulceration as part of the stress response
- Coagulopathy due to disseminated intravascular coagulation and hypothermia
- Haemolysis leading to haemoglobinuria and anaemia

Describe the principles behind the early management.

Immediate and early management of burns involves adherence to the ATLS system of trauma care involving identification of any other injuries

- Airway and Breathing: Looking for the presence of respiratory distress, which may not be in evidence initially. High flow oxygen is given. May require early intubation and ventilation
- Circulation: Monitoring of fluid therapy and cardiovascular function necessitates the insertion of a central venous catheter. The arterial pressure is supported with fluids
- Renal support involves the maintenance of the renal perfusion pressure with i.v. fluids. Given the added risk

of rhabdomyolysis, a urinary catheter should be inserted, and the urine output maintained >1 ml/kg/h

- Analgesia: using i.v. opioids or inhaled 70% nitrous oxide
- Prevention of hypothermia with convection heaters and a warm ambient temperature. This also helps to control the hypermetabolic state
- Stress ulcer prophylaxis is commenced
- Prophylactic antibiotic use is controversial, and should only be used for proven sepsis
- Surgery has a role in the emergency management of constricting circumferential thoracic eschars that can cause respiratory embarrassment
- Nutritional supplementation (preferably by the enteral route) should be commenced at an early stage

How much fluid would you give?

There are a number of formulae available to determine the rate and level of fluid replacement. However, ultimately the amount of fluid given depends on the clinical situation.

- i.v. fluids are commenced if >15% adult or >10% paediatric burns
- Deeper and more extensive burns may require a blood transfusion, especially in the context of other injuries
- The ATLS guideline is 2–4 ml/kg/% burn in the first 24 h, half of this to be given in the first 8 h
- The Mount Vernon formula divides fluid administration into a number of discrete time periods. The amount of fluid given in each period is the product of the weight and the % burn divided by two. The first 24 h is divided into periods of 4, 4, 4, 6, 6 and 12 h
- Crystalloid or colloid may be used. None has a proven survival benefit over the other

How do you assess the adequacy of fluid therapy?

A number of clinical parameters may be used.

- Clinical measures of the cardiac index: peripheral warmth capillary refill time and urine output

- Core temperature
- Haematocrit: determined by plasma volume and the red cell mass. Unreliable if there has been a recent transfusion or haemolysis
- Central venous pressure and its response to fluid challenges

CALCIUM BALANCE

What is the normal level of serum calcium?
2.2–2.6 mmol/l.

What is the distribution of calcium in the body?
99% of calcium is found in the bone – almost all as hydroxy-apatite. A small amount is readily exchangeable as calcium phosphate salts.

In what state is calcium found in the circulation?
- 50% is unbound and ionised
- 45% bound to plasma proteins
- 5% associated with anions such as citrate and lactate

Which organ systems are involved in controlling serum calcium levels?
The main organ systems are the gut, the kidneys and the skeletal system.

Name the hormones involved in controlling serum calcium.
Major hormones are
- *Parathormone (PTH):* of 84 amino acids, produced by the parathyroid glands
- *Vitamin D₃ (cholecalciferol) metabolites:* this is obtained via the diet and from the skin by conversion of 7-dehydrocholesterol
- *Calcitonin:* a 32 amino acid molecule produced by the thyroid's parafollicular (C) cells
- others, e.g. parathormone-related peptide

Briefly describe their effects.
- *PTH:* In the bone, increases the synthesis of enzymes that breakdown the matrix to release calcium and phosphate

▼

into the circulation. Also stimulates osteocytic and osteoclastic activity. Thus leads to progressive bone resorption. At the kidney, increases renal phosphate excretion, while reducing renal calcium loss. It also stimulates 1–α hydroxylase activity in the kidney, thus indirectly increasing calcium absorption

- *Vitamin D_3 metabolites:* The active metabolite is $1,25(OH)_2 D_3$ formed by renal hydroxylation of $25(OH)D_3$. This acts to increase the serum calcium while increasing the calcification of bone matrix. It acts on the bone to stimulate osteoblast proliferation and protein synthesis. At the kidney, it promotes calcium and phosphate reabsorption. It also enhances gut absorption of calcium and phosphate

- *Calcitonin:* This act to reduce the serum calcium if the level rises above 2.5 mmol/l. This inhibits bone resorption through inhibition of osteoclast activity. At the kidney, it stimulates the excretion of sodium, chloride, calcium and phosphate

What are the clinical consequences of hypercalcaemia?

- Renal calculi due to hypercalcinuria
- Nephrocalcinosis with multifocal calcium deposits in the renal parenchyma
- Increased gastric acid secretion stimulated by both calcium and PTH. Leads to dyspepsia and peptic ulceration
- Increased risk of acute pancreatitis
- Constipation
- Bone lesions: notably bone cysts, osteitis fibrosa cystica and Brown's tumours of bone
- Impairment of tubular function leads to polyuria and polydipsia. This can lead to dehydration, especially if there is associated vomiting
- Tiredness, lethargy and organic psychosis. In severe cases, leads to coma

C

What ECG changes may be found?

The ECG changes are related to alterations in the membrane potential and cardiac conduction. They are

- Shortened QT interval
- Increased PR interval, progressing to heart block
- Flattened or inverted T waves

Under which circumstances may a surgeon encounter a patient with hypercalcaemia?

The main reasons why a surgeon may encounter a hyper-calcaemic patient are

- Hypercalcaemia of malignancy, e.g. bronchogenic carcinoma, pathological fractures due to secondary deposits
- Primary hyperparathyroidism due to an adenoma of the parathyroid gland, requiring neck exploration
- In the context of hypercalcaemic complications, e.g. renal calculi, pancreatitis, peptic ulceration
- Renal transplant patient with tertiary hyperparathyroidism

What are the differential diagnoses of abdominal pain in the hypercalcaemic patient?

- Peptic ulceration with or without perforation
- Renal colic from calculi
- Acute pancreatitis
- Constipation from reduced intestinal motility

What does the emergency management of hypercalcaemia involve?

Management of acute hypercalcaemia (3.0–3.5 mmol/l) involves:

- Identifying and treating the underlying cause
- Commencing cardiac monitoring

▼

- Providing adequate rehydration with crystalloid. To prevent overload, central venous pressure (CVP) monitoring is required. Furosemide can be added to help in the calcium diuresuis
- A bisphosphonate infusion can rapidly reduce the serum calcium, e.g. pamidronate
- Calcitonin has a shorter duration of action, and is seldom used
- High dose steroids, e.g. prednisolone are useful in some cases, such as myeloma or sarcoidosis
- Urgent surgery is required in those cases due to hyperparathyroidism

What is the most important surgical cause of hypocalcaemia?

The most important surgical cause is after thyroid surgery when there is inadvertent removal of the parathyroid glands.

Give some of the recognised features of hypocalcaemia.

The important clinical features are
- Neuromuscular irritability manifest as peripheral and circumoral paraesthesia
- Muscular cramps
- Tetany
- *Chvostek's sign:* twitching of the facial muscles on tapping of the facial nerve
- *Trousseau's sign:* tetanic spasm of the hand following blood pressure cuff-induced arm ischaemia

What is the emergency management of hypocalcaemia?

- Commencement of cardiac monitoring
- Adequate fluid resuscitation
- 10 ml of 10% calcium gluconate is given initially, followed by 10–40 ml in a saline infusion over 4–8 h

CARDIAC ASSESSMENT

Give some examples of non-invasive investigations of cardiac function.

- *Pulse:* rate, rhythm, volume and character
- *Blood pressure using a pressure cuff:* measuring the absolute values, mean, and pulse pressure
- *ECG recording:* rate rhythm, intervals, axis and waveforms
- *Trans-thoracic echocardiography:* measuring systolic function, cardiac filling and valve function general morphology and blood flow
- Indicators of the cardiac index and peripheral organ perfusion
  - *Level of consciousness:* marker of cerebral perfusion
  - *Peripheral capillary refill*
  - *Urine output:* also a marker of renal function as well as cardiac function

Which invasive investigations do you know, and what information do they provide?

- *Blood pressure monitoring with arterial line:* exhibits a continuous arterial waveform and beat to beat variation
- *CVP monitoring with central line:* measuring the absolute value of the CVP or its response to fluid challenges and inotropes. The waveform may also be displayed continuously on a monitor
- *Pulmonary artery flotation catheter:* providing both direct and derived measures of left heart function. Also measures other parameters of cardiovascular function, such as systemic and pulmonary vascular resistance, and oxygen delivery/demand
- *Trans-oesophageal echocardiography:* Gives a more detailed picture of the left heart and thoracic aorta than trans–thoracic echo

▼

- Markers of the cardiac index and peripheral organ perfusion:
  - *Blood gases:* to assess the acidosis and base excess associated with anaerobic metabolism following poor tissue perfusion
  - *Serum lactate:* rising levels indicate a poor cardiac index
  - *Gastric tonometry:* Adequacy of splanchnic perfusion is estimated from gastric intramucosal pH measurements using a gastric probe. This is based on the belief that the gut is the first organ system to reflect a poor peripheral perfusion
  - *Mixed venous oxygen saturation (SvO$_2$):* Using a pulmonary artery catheter. A fall of the SvO$_2$ is suggestive of a fall in the cardiac output
  - *Arterial-venous oxygen difference:* This is increased in cases of poor organ perfusion where relative stagnation of blood leads to greater oxygen extraction

CARDIOGENIC SHOCK

What are the complications of myocardial infarction?

- *Cardiogenic shock*

- *Arrhythmias:* of ventricular or atrial origin, resulting in tachy- or bradycardia. Heart block may also ensue. The type of arrhythmia depends on the extent and territory of the infarct

- *Mechanical complications:*
  - *Ventricular septal defect (VSD):* complicates 1 in 200 infarcts. Result is acute right heart volume overload and pulmonary oedema
  - *Free wall rupture,* which may result in pericardial tamponade
  - *Papillary muscle rupture,* presenting as acute mitral or tricuspid regurgitation
  - *Left ventricular aneurysm* with mural thrombus. This may be a late presentation with progressive cardiac failure or systemic embolism (leading to stroke or acute limb/mesenteric infarction). There is persistent S-T segment elevation

- *Pericarditis as part of Dressler's syndrome:* may occur several weeks after infarction with chest pain and pyrexia. Thought to be due to an immunological process

- *Chronic cardiac failure:* long term deterioration in ventricular function as part of the on-going ischaemic process

What is the definition of cardiogenic shock?

Cardiogenic shock is defined as inadequate tissue perfusion resulting directly from myocardial dysfunction. Cardiac index is less than 2.2l/min/m^2 with a pulmonary artery occlusion pressure of $>16 \text{mmHg}$ and a systolic pressure of $<90 \text{mmHg}$.

The resulting tissue hypoxia persists despite adequate intravascular volume replacement.

Mention some of the causes of cardiogenic shock.

The main causes are

- Following a large myocardial infarction with resulting abnormal ventricular wall motion and systolic dysfunction

- *Acute cardiac arrhythmias:* tachyarrhythmias can lead to shortened diastolic filling time with reduced cardiac output. Bradyarrhythmias lead to a direct fall in the cardiac output

- *Post cardiac surgery and prolonged cardiopulmonary bypass:* this can lead to myocardial 'stunning' which is a temporary reduction in the cardiac output despite restoration of myocardial perfusion. This occurs due to metabolic changes in the myocytes brought on by cardioplegic arrest, producing a low output state

- *Following infection:* severe viral myocarditis can lead to systolic dysfunction. Also, infective endocarditis can produce valve rupture with acute incompetence

- *Cardiac trauma:* resulting in a myocardial contusion

What are the clinical features of cardiogenic shock, and how may it be distinguished from other causes of shock?

The clinical features are

- Evidence of reduced cardiac index (cardiac output per m^2 body surface area):
  - Cool peripheries
  - Reduced capillary return
  - Reduced urine output
  - Reduced level of consciousness from poor cerebral perfusion
- Elevated venous pressure:
  - Pulmonary oedema
  - Elevated jugular venous pulse
  - Hepatomegaly from hepatic engorgement

- Reduced arterial pressure: typically a systolic pressure of ≤90 mmHg
- On auscultation: gallop rhythm of a third heart sound. Also fourth heart sound may be in evidence. An associated bruit may reveal the underlying cause, e.g. VSD or mitral regurgitation

It may be difficult to distinguish clinically from the shock of cardiac tamponade or pulmonary embolism. However, in cardiogenic shock, the dominant feature is the presence of acute pulmonary oedema.

In septic shock, the cardiac output is initially increased, with presence of bounding pulses and warm peripheries following a fall in the systemic vascular resistance. The JVP is not elevated.

What is the pathophysiology of decompensating cardiogenic shock?

This may be summarised by the following diagram:

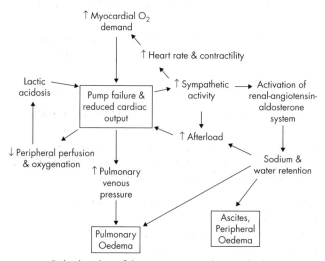

Pathophysiology of decompensating cardiogenic shock

The basis for the pathophysiology lies at the Frank–Starling curve. The curve is shifted to the right, reflecting a higher end-diastolic pressure and volume to achieve the same stroke volume. The compensatory increase in the heart rate and contractility arising from sympathetic activity also leads to increased myocardial oxygen demand. Note that progressive lactic acidosis suppresses myocardial contractility directly.

Which investigations are useful for cardiogenic shock?

The following special investigations are useful in establishing the diagnosis and severity of the cardiogenic shock in the ITU

- ECG: for the presence of infarction or arrhythmia
- CXR
- Echocardiogram: trans-thoracic and trans-oesophageal forms may be performed at the bedside
- Pulmonary artery catheterisation

What changes can be seen on the plain P-A chest radiograph?

- *Increased cardiothoracic ratio:* reflecting a dilated, volume overloaded ventricle

- *Kerley B lines:* short-line shadows above the costophrenic angle. They reflect interstitial oedema of the septa

- *Interstitial shadowing* of pulmonary oedema

- *Hilar 'bat's wing' shadowing* further evidence of oedema

- *Prominent upper lobe pulmonary vessels* indicating venous congestion

- *Left atrial enlargement* seen as double shadowing at the atrial position, or prominence at the left heart border (due to enlargement of the left atrial appendage)

What information can be obtained from an echocardiogram?

This provide the following information

- Anatomic information, such as the presence of valve lesions or a VSD

- Colour flow may be added to allow quantification of flow across a valve or septal defect. From this pressure differences can be gleamed
- The ventricular contractility and function can be calculated from end-systolic and end-diastolic measurements
- Note that by virtue of its position, trans-oesophageal echocardiography provides a better picture of the left atrium and valve function

What are the findings from the pulmonary artery catheter in cardiogenic shock?

- Elevated central venous pressure
- Cardiac index of $<2.2\,l/min/m^2$
- Pulmonary artery occlusion pressure of $>16\,mmHg$
- Decreased mixed venous oxygen saturation

CENTRAL LINE INSERTION

C

What is CVP and how may it be determined?

This is the pressure in the right atrium (right atrial filling pressure).

It may be estimated clinically by examining the jugular venous pulse at the root of the neck, or measured directly by central venous cannulation.

What is the normal value for the CVP?

0–10 mmHg or 0–8 cmH$_2$O.

How useful is it as a measure of the circulating volume?

The absolute value of the CVP in determining filling is not as useful as its response to a 200–300 ml fluid challenge over 1–3 min (*see* below).

In some critically ill (mainly cardiac and pulmonary diseases) where the myocardial compliance is affected, or in cases of valvular heart disease, the CVP reading provides an inaccurate estimate of the volume state. Thus, the reading has to be interpreted in the light of other physiological parameters.

Draw the three types of response to fluid challenge.

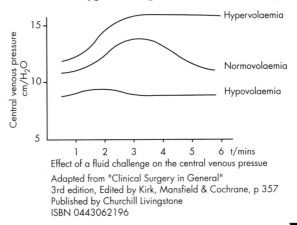

Effect of a fluid challenge on the central venous pressue

Adapted from "Clinical Surgery in General"
3rd edition, Edited by Kirk, Mansfield & Cochrane, p 357
Published by Churchill Livingstone
ISBN 0443062196

What are the uses of the central venous cannula?

Central venous lines have both short- and long-term uses:

- Short-term:
  - CVP measurements
  - Pulmonary artery catheterisation providing various direct and derived measures of cardiovascular function
  - Fluid resuscitation
  - Drug administration: for toxic or irritant drugs, such as amiodarone, potassium or inotropes
  - Haemodialysis
  - Transvenous cardiac pacing
- Long-term:
  - Venous blood sampling in the long-term, e.g. Hickman lines
  - Drug administration: such as cytotoxics
  - Feeding by the use of total parenteral nutrition

To reduce infection risk, these lines may be tunneled beneath the skin for a distance before entering the vein. Also, patency is ensured by regular heparin–saline flushes.

What is the 'Seldinger technique'?

This is a technique of cannulation that involves the use of a guide wire passed through an introducing-needle. A wider bore cannula is then passed over the wire after removal of the introducing-needle. Finally, the wire is removed. These principles can also be applied to other procedures, such as paracentesis or percutaneous tracheostomy.

Which vessels may be used for central access?

- Internal jugular vein (most common)
- Subclavian vein
- Femoral vein
- Less commonly, the axilliary, cephalic or external jugular veins

Which surface landmarks define the course of the internal jugular vein and the superior vena cava?

The internal jugular vein runs from the lobule of the ear to the medial end of the clavicle, where it lies between the two heads of the sternocleidomastoid muscle. Behind the sterno-clavicular joint, it unites with the subclavian vein to form the right brachiocephalic vein.

This joins the left brachiocephalic behind the right 1st costal cartilage to form the superior vena cava. This passes vertically down and pierces the pericardium at the level of the 2nd costal cartilage, entering the right atrium behind the 3rd costal cartilage.

Where is the point of entry of the needle for internal jugular and subclavian venous access?

- Internal jugular cannulation
  - The patient is placed in the Trendelenberg (head down) position
  - The vein may be approached as it lies deep to the two heads of the sternocleidomastoid
  - The needle is directed inferiorly parallel to the sagittal plane, at 30° to the skin
- Subclavian vein cannulation
  - The approach is infraclavicular
  - The point of entry is 2 cm below the mid-point of the clavicle
  - The needle is directed deep to the clavicle, pointing to the jugular notch

For both methods, the skin is prepared and locally anaes-thetised. The Seldinger method is employed for cannulation. A chest radiograph is taken at the end of the procedure to ensure a correct position and exclude a pneumo/haemothorax.

Describe some complications of central line insertion.

Complications may be described in relation to surrounding structures

- Pleural complications
  - Pneumothorax
- Venous complications
  - Air embolism
  - Thrombosis (more common with the femoral route)
- Arterial complications
  - Inadvertent cannulation
  - Local haematoma
  - Exsanguination (subclavian artery injury is difficult to control)
  - Haemothorax
- Lymphatic complications
  - Thoracic duct injury can lead to a chylothorax
- Cardiac complications
  - Right atrial perforation leading to cardiac tamponade
  - Arrhythmias: ECG monitoring is mandatory during cannulation
- Localised or generalised sepsis (initiated at insertion)

In which two ways may the information from a central line be presented?

As a continuous waveform using a transducer attached to an oscilloscope, or intermittently by the use of a manometer system at the bedside.

Which formula governs the rate of flow through tubes, and how does this affect the use of a central line in fluid resuscitation?

Flow through can be defined in terms of the Hagen–Poiseuille formula that states that

$$\text{Flow through a rigid tube} = \frac{P\,r^4\,\pi}{8\eta L}$$

where P = driving pressure; r = tube radius; η = viscosity; L = tube length.

Thus, the greatest flow can be achieved with short, wide tubes. The radius of the tube has the greatest impact since the flow is proportional to the fourth power of the radius. Central lines are not the most effective for rapid fluid administration because of their length and radius.

$$Flow = radius^4$$

CHRONIC RENAL FAILURE

What is the difference between creatinine and creatine?

Creatinine is creatine minus a water molecule (i.e. the anhydride of creatine). It is formed in muscle by the non-enzymatic and irreversible degradation of creatine phosphate.

Creatine is an amino acid derivative formed from methionine, glycine and arginine, and stored in muscle and brain tissue. During periods of low muscular activity, it is phosphorylated by ATP into creatine phosphate. When muscle activity increases, creatine phosphate delivers this phosphate back to ADP, releasing creatine and ATP. Thus, creatine acts as a ready and direct source of high energy phosphate groups for muscle contraction.

What, then, is creatine kinase?

Creatine kinase is the enzyme that is involved in the donation of phosphate to creatine from ATP, forming creatine phosphate.

What is the normal level of serum creatinine?

60–120 μmol/L. Note that the units are given as μmols and not mmols.

Why is the serum creatinine a better indicator of renal function than serum urea concentration?

Serum urea is a poorer indicator of the glomerular filtration rate (GFR) than creatinine, since 50% or so of the filtered urea undergoes reabsorption at the tubules, leading to an underestimation of the GFR. Also, the daily production of urea is more variable than creatinine.

What is the incidence of chronic renal failure?

The incidence is 600 per 100,000 of the population per year in the UK.

▼

Give some causes for chronic renal failure.

The causes may be classified under a number of different headings

- *Congenital:*
  - Polycystic kidney disease
- *Glomerular disease:*
  - Chronic glomerulonephritis
  - Diabetes mellitus
  - Amyloidosis
- *Reno-vascular:*
  - Hypertensive nephrosclerosis
  - Chronic vasculitis, e.g. SLE
- *Tubular/interstitial:*
  - Chronic interstitial nephritis
  - Chronic pyelonephritis
- *Chronic outflow obstruction:*
  - Calculi
  - Prostatic enlargement
  - Pelvic tumours

How may polycystic kidneys present?

They may present with loin pain, haematuria, pyelonephritis or hypertension. The extra-renal manifestations may, on occasion, be the first indication. (see below)

Other than renal failure, what are the complications of polycystic kidneys?

The extra-renal manifestations are

- Cysts in other organs: liver, pancreas, spleen, ovaries
- Berry aneurysms at the circle of Willis: increased risk of subarachnoid haemorrhage
- Mitral valve prolapse

C

What are the clinical features and complications of chronic renal failure?

Clinical signs and symptoms may not be seen until the GFR is <15% of normal:

- *Hypertension*

- *Polyuria and nocturia:* due to the osmotic diuresis caused by uraemia

- *Oedema:* due to a combination of fluid retention and proteinuria

- *Features of uraemia:* due to circulating 'uraemic toxins' such as organic acids. Leads to skin pigmentation, anorexia, nausea, malaise and constipation

- *Anaemia:* normocytic and normochromic. Leads to lethargy and dyspnoea

- *Renal osteodystrophy:* A combination of osteomalacia, osteitis fibrosa cystica and osteosclerosis. Leads to a secondary hyperparathyroidism. Can lead to metastatic calcification, bone pain and pathological fractures

- *Neurological:* myoclonic twitches, muscle cramps, mental slowing

Some complications are

- *Cardiac:* uraemic cardiomyopathy

- *Pericardial:* uraemic pericarditis

- *Vascular:* peripheral vascular disease due to a combination of hyperlipidaemia and hypertension

- *Pulmonary oedema*

- *Bony complications* mentioned above

- *Bleeding tendency:* due to platelet dysfunction

Run through the list of acid–base and electrolyte disturbances seen.

- Hyponatraemia
- Hyperkalaemia
- Hypocalcaemia

- Hyperphosphataemia
- Metabolic acidosis
- Reduced serum bicarbonate
- Increased serum creatinine

What is the pathophysiology of renal osteodystrophy?

There are a number of pathological processes that lead to bone disease:

- There is a reduction of renal production of 1-α hydroxylase resulting in a reduction of calcitriol (1,25 (OH)$_2$ D$_3$)
- This leads to a secondary hyperparathyroidism
- There is also hyperphosphataemia as a direct consequence of reduced renal function
- Hyperparathyroidism produces increased bone resorption, bone cyst formation and osteitis fibrosa cystica
- Deficiency of 1,25 (OH)$_2$ D$_3$ reduces bone mineralisation with resulting osteomalacia

Why are uraemic patients anaemic?

Uraemic patients may develop a normocytic, normochromic anaemia for a number of reasons:

- Deficiency of erythropoietin – the most important cause
- Presence of circulating bone marrow toxins
- Bone marrow fibrosis during osteitis fibrosa cystica
- Increased red cell fragility caused by uraemic toxins

What would you expect to find when examining a patient with chronic renal failure?

- The patient may be tachypnoeic from metabolic acidosis
- Pigmentation of the skin as a direct effect of uraemia. There may also be scratch marks on the skin from uraemic pruritis
- Hands: brown discolouration in the fingernails, or a fistula at the wrist for dialysis
- Abdomen: may reveal the scar from a previous renal transplant

- Cardiovascular: hypertension due to fluid retention. There may be a pericardial friction rub from uraemic pericarditis. Peripherally, pitting oedema is common
- Peripheral neuropathy also develops
- Features of the underlying cause: palpable kidneys in polycystic disease, peripheral vascular disease in diabetes mellitus

How is chronic renal failure managed?

The principles of management are

- Management of bone disease: to improve bone mineralisation and hypocalcaemia, patients are given α-calcidol and calcitriol (1,25 $(OH)_2$ D_3). Hyperphosphataemia can be managed with the use of gut phosphate binders such as calcium chloride. Aluminium compounds have also been used, but they can lead to bone disease themselves, and dementia
- Anaemia can be reversed with the use of subcutaneous recombinant human erythropoeitin
- Hypertension: generally managed with the same agents as those with normal renal function. High dose loop diuretics are in common use
- Dietary considerations: protein intake is restricted to 40 g/day to reduce urea production. Sodium restriction helps to limit fluid overload. Potassium restriction is also required. Vitamin supplements replace the water-soluble vitamins lost during dialysis
- Fluid restriction limits the development of oedema
- Other aspects of management: control of nausea, laxatives for constipation
- End-stage renal failure requires haemodialysis or renal transplantation

COAGULATION DEFECTS

What are the basic components to normal haemostatic function?

Normal haemostatic function depends on the normal inter-play of a number of components

- Normal vascular endothelial function and tissue integrity
- Normal platelet number and function
- Normal amounts of the coagulation factors and their normal function
- Presence of various essential agents, such as vitamin K and calcium
- Balanced relationship between the fibrinolytic pathway and the clotting cascade

What do platelets do, and what is their origin?

Platelets have a number of functions during the haemostatic response

- *Vasoconstriction:* during the platelet release reaction, vasoactive mediators such as serotonin, thromboxane A2 and ADP are released

- *Factor-binding:* platelet membrane phospholipid, through a reaction involving calcium and vitamin K, binds to factors II, VII, IX, and X. This serves to concentrate and co-ordinate factors into the same area for maximum activation

- *Formation of the primary haemostatic plug:* further stabilised by platelet granule enzymes

Platelets are formed in the bone marrow and released by megakaryocyte fragmentation.

What is von Willebrand's factor?

von Willebrand factor is a molecule synthesised by megakaryocytes and endothelial cells. It facilitates the binding of platelets to the sub-endothelial connective tissue, and binds to factor VIII.

What is the function of vitamin K?

Vitamin K, a fat-soluble vitamin, is involved in the pathway that leads to factors II, VII, IX and X binding to the surface of platelets. Specifically, it is involved in the carboxylation of these factors which allows them to bind to calcium, and hence the surface of platelets.

Which factors are involved in the intrinsic pathway?

The factor and co-factors of the intrinsic system are VIII, IX, X, XI and XII.

Which factors are involved in the extrinsic pathway?

The factors and co-factors of the extrinsic pathway are tissue factor, factors VII and X.

What is the end result of the coagulation cascade?

The end product of the coagulation cascade is the formation of a stable meshwork of cross-linked fibrin around the primary platelet plug. This therefore forms the stable haemostatic plug.

Give some reasons why a surgical patient may develop a coagulopathy.

Causes of a coagulopathy in the surgical patient include

- *Hypothermia:* a cold patient has dysfunctioning platelets

- *Massive blood transfusion:* packed red cells do not contain platelets, so a large transfusion leads to a dilutional loss. Also, stored blood rapidly loses the function of the labile factors V and VIII

- *Aspirin therapy:* those with cardiovascular disease may be on aspirin prior to surgery. This leads to reduced platelet function by interfering with thromboxane A2 synthesis

- *Heparin therapy:* this not only directly interferes with clotting, but leads to thrombocytopenia through an immunologic mechanism – the so-called 'heparin-induced thrombocytopenia syndrome' or 'HITS'

- *Dextran infusions* also affect platelet and coagulation factor function
- *Sepsis:* a cause of DIC
- Development of *post-operative acute renal or liver failure*

How may a coagulopathy be recognised in the surgical patient?

- Persisting small vessel bleeding intraoperatively, despite achieving adequate surgical haemostasis
- Post-operative bleeding: excess blood loss from the drains
- Platelet problems presenting as a new-onset purpuric rash
- Bleeding from unusual areas: venepuncture or cannulation sites, epistaxis, haematuria from uncomplicated bladder catheterisation

Which tests are used to investigate the coagulopathies?

- The platelet count
- Tests of platelet function:
  - Bleeding time (range 3–8 min)
  - Adhesion studies: e.g. with epinephrine, collagen or ristocetin
- Prothrombin time: (9–15 s): a measure of the extrinsic and common pathways and the degree of warfarinisation
- Activated partial thromboplastin time: (30–40 s): a measure of the intrinsic and common pathways. Also a measure of heparin therapy
- Thrombin time (14–16 s): a measure of the final common pathway
- Individual factor assay
- Fibrin-degradation products: when testing for DIC

DISSEMINATED INTRAVASCULAR COAGULATION (DIC)

What is the basic pathophysiology of DIC?

There is pathological activation of the coagulation pathway by damaged tissues that release cytokines and tissue factors. This is followed by pathologic activation of the fibrinolytic pathway. This has a number of effects

- Diffuse intravascular thrombosis leading to small and large vessel occlusion by fibrin
- Vascular occlusion leads to shock and end organ failure
- Bleeding tendency with consumption of clotting factors and platelets
- This manifests itself as bleeding from mucosal surfaces and a petechial rash
- If presenting as shock, there is a low cardiac index and hypotension despite tachycardia
- Patients may therefore develop renal failure and acute respiratory distress syndrome

How may DIC be triggered?

- Infections: particularly gram negative or anaerobic sepsis, or viral sources such as HIV, CMV or hepatitis
- Trauma-related:
  - Multiple trauma
  - Burns
  - Hypothermia
- Malignancy: leads to chronic DIC
- Transfusion reaction
- Obstetric causes:
  - Amniotic fluid embolism
  - Placental abruption
  - Eclampsia
- Liver failure

What type of anaemia may be seen in DIC and why?

Microangiopathic haemolytic anaemia may be seen due to red cell fragmentation caused by fibrin deposition in vessel walls. It can be seen on blood film examination.

What will haematologic investigations show in cases of DIC?

- D-dimer: this is a fibrin–degradation product, elevation of which indicates activation of the fibrinolytic pathway
- Platelet count below 15×10^9/l: due to consumption with activation of the clotting cascade
- Decreased fibrinogen
- Abnormal clotting screen: with a rise in the PT and the APTT in the acute situation
- Reduction in the individual clotting factors

Which blood products are used in the management of DIC?

Platelets and FFP are used to replenish the consumed factors. Packed red cells may also be required if the haemolytic anaemia is severe enough.

D

DISSEMINATED INTRAVASCULAR COAGULATION

ECG I – BASIC CONCEPTS

Where are the anatomic locations of the sino–atrial and atrioventricular (AV) nodes?

The sino-atrial node is an elliptical area found at the junction of the superior vena cava and the right atrium.

The atrioventricular node is found in a triangular area of the right atrial wall just above the septal cusp of the tricuspid valve.

Where on the body are the ECG leads placed?

The locations of the electrodes are

- Bipolar leads: attached to the right arm, left arm and left leg
- Unipolar (chest) leads
  - V1: 4th interspace, right of sternum
  - V2: 4th interspace, left of sternum
  - V3: Midway between V2 & V4
  - V4: Normal apex (left 5th interspace, mid–clavicular line)
  - V5: Anterior axillary line at the level of V4
  - V6: Mid-axillary line at the level of V4

Draw a typical ECG waveform, and label the various deflections.

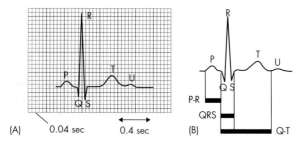

(A) Normal ECG complexes. (B) P-R, QRS and QT segments.

P-R Interval: 0.12–0.20s QRS Interval <0.12s QTc 0.35–0.43s

Diagram from "Cardiology" by Julian & Cowan 6th ed. p 14
Published by Baillière Tindall
ISBN 0702016446

E

When do the heart sounds occur in relation to the electrical cycle of the heart?

The first heart sound (following closure of the atrioventricular valves) is heard at the end of the R wave on the ECG. The second heart sound (following closure of the ventriculoarterial valves) is heard at the end of the T wave on the ECG (*see* illustration).

What is the origin of the P wave?

The P wave deflection is caused by the passage of current through the atrium. Note that it is not due to electrical activity at the sinoatrial node, which is not shown in the ECG recording.

Define the PR interval. What does it represent, and what is the normal range?

The PR interval is measured from the beginning of the P wave to the beginning of the QRS complex. It corresponds to the time taken for the impulse to travel from the sinoatrial node to the ventricle. In adults, the normal range is 0.12–0.20 s.

What does the QRS interval represent, and what is the upper limit of its duration?

The QRS complex represents ventricular muscle depolarisation and the upper limit is 0.12 s.

Define the QT interval.

The QT interval is from the start of the QRS complex to the end of the T wave. It represents the time from the onset of ventricular depolarisation to full repolarisation. Its duration is heart rate-dependant.

What is the QTc interval, and how is it calculated?

The QTc interval is the QT interval that has been corrected for variations in the heart rate. It represents the QT interval

▼

standardised to a heart rate of 60 beats per minute, and permits comparisons between and within individuals.

It is calculated by Bazett's formula

$$\frac{QT\ interval}{\sqrt{RR\ interval}}$$

It follows that at a heart rate of 60, the QT = QTc. The normal range is 0.35–0.43 s.

What does the T wave represent, and why is its deflection in the same direction as the QRS complex?

The T wave represents <u>ventricular myocardial repolarisation</u>. Since it represents repolarisation, one would expect the deflection to be negative. However, repolarisation takes place from the epicardium to endocardium, which is the opposite direction to depolarisation. Thus, causing the deflection to be in the same direction as for depolarisation.

Have you heard of J and U waves? Where in the electrical cycle may they appear, and under what circumstances may they be seen?

J wave: The J-point of the normal ECG is found at the junction of the S wave and the ST segment. <u>A J wave</u> is a upward deflection found at this point, and may be seen in <u>hypothermia</u>.

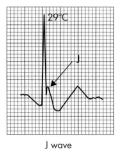

J wave

Diagram from "Cardiology" by Julian & Cowan 6th ed. p 24
Published by Baillière Tindall
ISBN 0702016446

U wave: This is a low voltage wave found after the T wave of some normal individuals, but can become more prominent in cases of hypokalaemia.

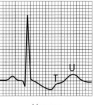

U wave

Diagram from "Cardiology" by Julian & Cowan 6th ed. p 23
Published by Baillière Tindall
ISBN 0702016446

ECG II – RATE AND RHYTHM DISTURBANCES

Give some causes of sinus tachycardia.
- Exercise
- Pain and anxiety
- Pyrexia
- Shock of any cause
- Hyperthyroidism
- Anaemia
- Drugs: Catacholamines, atropine, aminophylline

Give some causes of sinus bradycardia.
- Athletes Heart
- Hypothyroidism
- Raised intracranial pressure (as part of the Cushing reflex)
- Jaundice
- Drugs: β-blockers, digoxin

What kinds of supraventricular arrhythmias do you know?
- Atrial ectopics
- Supraventricular tachycardia
- Atrial flutter and fibrillation

What are the characteristic features of a supraventricular tachycardia?
- A heart rate in the order of 150–220 beats per minute
- The QRS complex duration is within normal limits
- P waves may be of abnormal shape, or absent altogether
- May be difficult to distinguish from atrial flutter with 2:1 block

How are attacks managed?

Paroxysms may be terminated through simple measures to stimulate vagal activity, such as the valsalva manoeuvre, or carotid sinus massage. Alternatively, by the use of i.v. adenosine, which transiently blocks AV conduction. Verapamil has also been used.

What are the characteristic features of atrial flutter?

- Rapid tachycardia an atrial rate of 250–350 beats per minute
- ECG shows 'sawtooth'-shape flutter waves
- Often seen with variable degrees of AV block, e.g. 2:1, 3:1 or 4:1
- The ventricular rate is correspondingly less in cases seen with AV block
- QRS complexes are of normal morphology

What is the relationship of atrial flutter with atrial fibrillation?

Although these two types of arrhythmias are distinct entities, they may co-exist in the same patient. Atrial flutter may also progress to atrial fibrillation.

What triggers atrial flutter?

Atrial flutter is often triggered by the presence of organic cardiac disease, such as post-rheumatic fever, ischaemic heart disease, valve disease or myocarditis.

What are the basic principles of management of cardiac arrhythmias?

- *Chemical cardioversion:* e.g. amiodarone in atrial fibrillation
- *Electrical cardioversion:* for use in cases of atrial fibrillation and ventricular tachycardia

- *Induction of AV conduction delay:* Adenosine for SVT, or digoxin providing rate control in cases of atrial fibrillation

- *Cardiac pacing:* either temporarily or permanently, as in heartblock

- *Ablation of arrhythmia source,* either at cardiac catheterisation, or surgically

Draw basic rhythm strips of hearts exhibiting 1st degree, 2nd and complete AV block, identifying the defining morphology.

1st degree block: A prolonged PR interval that is fixed in duration.

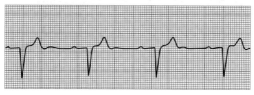

1st Degree Heart Block
- Prolonged P-R Interval
- Constant in timing
- Always followed by a QRS complex

2nd degree block:
- *Mobitz I (Wenkebach phenomena):* The PR interval becomes progressively more prolonged, until one of the P waves is not followed by a QRS complex. After this, the cycle repeats itself

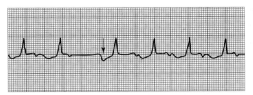

2nd Degree Block
Mobitz I (Werckebach) Block
• Progressive lengthening of the P-R interval
• Until a P wave fails to be conducted

• *Mobitz II:* Some of the P waves are not followed by a QRS, and this is consistent between beats, e.g. 2:1, 3:1 etc

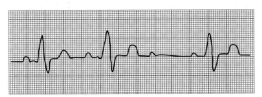

2nd Degree Heart Block
Mobitz II Block
P-R intervals normal & constant
But an occasional P wave is not conducted

3rd degree (complete) heart block: There is no recognisable relationship between the P waves and the onset of the QRS complexes.

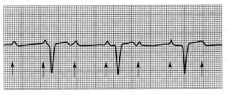

3rd Degree Block (complete)
P waves bear no relationship to the QRS complex
∴ Atria & Ventricles function independently

Diagram from "Cardiology" by Julian & Cowan 6th ed
Published by Baillière Tindall
ISBN 0702016446

What are the clinical features of complete heart block?

- Variable 1st heart sounds
- Cannon "a" waves in the JVP

How is a complete heart block managed?

With the use of a permanent pacemaker.

ENDOTRACHEAL INTUBATION

By which routes may the trachea be intubated?
Through the orotracheal and nasotracheal routes.

What are the indications for intubation?
Indications include
- For standard anaesthesia when using IPPV and muscle relaxation
- To provide airway protection from gastric contents which may be aspirated, e.g. in cases of severe head injury when ventilation is also required
- To permit airway suction
- Thoracic surgical procedures that require one-lung isolation. Here, there is endobronchial intubation to allow individual control of the lungs

What are the basic steps involved in intubation under general anaesthesia?
- Pre-oxygenation: where 100% oxygen is administered for 3–5 min
- Positioning: 'sniffing the morning air', with the head extended
- Anaesthesia: local (for awake intubation) or general. Muscle relaxation used with general anaesthetic
- Laryngoscopy
- Intubation
- Cuff inflation
- Connection to oxygen source
- Check correct position with auscultation of both lung fields
- Secure in place with tape

What is the purpose of pre-oxygenation prior to intubation?

The purpose is to increase the time to which the patient becomes hypoxaemic during intubation by increasing the PaO_2.

Name some pieces of equipment that may be used during intubation.

- Laryngoscope
- Tracheal tube
- Bougie: which can be used to guide the tube into the correct position
- Cotton tape to allow the tube to be secured
- 10 ml syringe to inflate the cuff with air
- Connector to attach the tube to the breathing system
- Stethoscope to check the correct position
- Suction device with cases of rapid-sequence induction

What is the difference between a Magill and Mcintosh laryngoscope?

The Magill is a straight-bladed instrument, and the Mcintosh has a curved blade.

In which anatomical position does the tip of the laryngoscope blade sit during adult and paediatric intubation?

In the adult, the tip of the blade is in the vallecula, anterior to the epiglottis. In children, the tip lies behind the epiglottis.

What shape of laryngoscope blade is used for paediatric anaesthesia and why?

A straight-bladed laryngoscope is used for paediatric intubation. In children, the epiglottis is floppy and U-shaped. The straight blade passes behind the epiglottis, fixing it in position, so that it can be lifted forward to expose the laryngeal opening.

▼

What are the main morphological differences between the airway of an adult and that of a child?

In children

- The tongue is relatively large
- The epiglottis is relatively larger and more U-shaped
- The larynx is higher up (at C3/4)
- The angle at the tracheal bifurcation (carina) is greater
- The right and left main bronchi come off the trachea at the same angle. In adults, the right main bronchus is more vertical
- The cricoid ring is the narrowest point of the laryngeal complex. In the adult, it is the glottis of the vocal folds

What common sizes of laryngeal tube are available for the adult?

Common sizes are 9.0–9.5 mm in males and 8.0–8.5 mm in females. The size refers to the internal diameter.

How is tube size calculated for the child?

The size of the tube in children is calculated by the formula

$$\frac{\text{Age}}{4} + 4\,\text{mm}$$

Is a general anaesthetic always required for intubation?

No, awake intubation is achieved with a local-anaesthetic throat spray or nerve block. Awake intubation is performed in those who are at risk of imminent airway obstruction if intubated with a general anaesthetic and muscle relaxation.

What is rapid sequence induction, and what important features define this form of intubation?

This is required for emergency induction of anaesthesia, where there is a risk of gastric aspiration. The important requirements are

- Skilled assistant
- Suction equipment at the ready

- Cricoid pressure applied by the assistant. It is released only when the cuff is inflated
- i.v. induction with suxamethonium to achieve rapid muscle relaxation

When is nasotracheal intubation performed?

- ENT procedures
- Oral surgery
- When long-term intubation is anticipated, since there is no interference with the mouth

What are the complications of endotracheal intubation?

- Trauma to upper-airway structures, e.g. teeth, pharynx, and larynx
- Spinal injury to those with an unstable neck, e.g. trauma, rheumatoid neck
- Acute hypertension upon laryngoscopy due to an autonomic reflex
- Laryngospasm or bronchospasm
- Gastric aspiration
- Misplaced tube, e.g. inadvertent bronchial intubation, oesophageal intubation
- Inadvertent extubation or disconnection from the gas supply
- Mucosal ulceration and tracheal stenosis

How long can the tube be left in place?

Generally, the tube is not left for greater than 2 weeks to prevent long-term complications. Tracheostomy may be performed if prolonged intubation is anticipated.

ENTERAL NUTRITION

What are the indications for enteral nutrition?

Enteral feeding should be provided for those patients with a functionally intact gastro-intestinal system that cannot meet their daily nutritional requirements.

By which routes may enteral nutrition be administered?

- *Oral nutritional supplementation:* these are taken between meals, being mainly milk or soya protein-based

- *Nasoenteric feeding:* either into the stomach (nasogastric, NG) or jejunum (nasojejunal, NJ) using a fine bore feeding tube to minimise oesophageal irritation.
  NJ feeding bypasses the stomach for those with impaired gastric motility and reduces pancreatic stimulation in those with pancreatitis. Therefore it has reduced the risk of pulmonary aspiration

- *Gastrostomy:* this may be placed during surgery or percutaneously by endoscopic or fluoroscopic techniques. It is suitable for prolonged feeding, particularly in those with head injuries or other neurological deficits affecting co-ordinated swallowing

- *Jejunostomy:* this is usually placed at laparotomy in those in whom prolonged feeding is anticipated. The tube is sutured to the antimesenteric side of the jejunum. Note that this bypasses the pancreas and biliary tree and reduces the risk of aspiration

What is the difference between a polymeric and elemental diet?

A polymeric diet is given to those with well functioning GI tracts, unlike elemental diets which are reserved for those with malabsorption, e.g. short bowel syndrome.

With polymeric diets, whole protein is used as the source of nitrogen, but for elemental, free amino acids or oligopeptides are used. Glucose polymers and long-chain triglycerides are the source of carbohydrate and fat respectively for elemental diets.

What other enteral diets are available?

- *Modular diets:* this diet has been enriched in a particular nutrient for the requirement of specific patients
- *Special formulation diets:* these are arranged for specific diseases, e.g. ventilated patients are given a diet rich in fat as the main energy source as opposed to glucose, in order to reduce CO_2 generation during metabolism

Why is it necessary to give gastrically fed patients a break from feeding at some point during a 24-hour period?

There are two main reasons why gastric feeding is not continuous:

- Feeding without a break encourages bacterial colonisation of the stomach. This increases the risk of a nosocomial pneumonia if there is aspiration
- Continuous intragastric feeding causes a secretory response from the ascending colon leading to diarrhoea. This may be due to the loss of the normal cephalic phase of secretion

What happens to the bowel in those who are not fed enterally?

It is known that absence of enteral feeding leads to atrophic changes in the intestinal mucosa. This is because local hormonal release in response to food stimulates the release of enzymes necessary for mucosal integrity.

What is the result of mucosal atrophy?

- Loss of cellular adhesion and development of cellular channels
- Translocation of bacteria across the bowel wall into the systemic circulation is encouraged. This can lead to sepsis,

▼

or perpetuation of the systemic inflammatory response in the critically ill

Give some complications associated with enteral feeding.

- Displacement of the tube: jejunal migration can lead to diarrhoea
- Infection around a gastrostomy or jejunostomy wound
- Refeeding syndrome: leads to hypophosphataemia in the malnourished, with thrombocytopenia and confusion
- Hyperkalaemia in those with renal impairment
- Hyperglycaemia in those with the reduced glucose tolerance of the critically ill

EXTUBATION AND WEANING

What are some of the prerequisites to successful extubation?

- The original disease process that leads to the requirement for ventilation must be resolved
- Lung function must be adequate
- No signs of sepsis: this increases the metabolic and respiratory demands, as well as increasing CO_2 production
- Haemodynamic stability
- Nutrition must be satisfactory
- The patients' mental state must be good enough to obey commands i.e. no confusion or agitation that may jeopardise success. This requires a progressive reversal of sedation

What is meant by 'adequate' lung function in this context?

Some satisfactory lung function parameters are

- Respiratory rate <35/min
- PaO_2 >11 kPa at an FiO_2 of <0.5
- Minute volume <10 l/min
- Vital capacity >10 ml/kg
- Tidal volume >5 ml/kg
- Maximum inspiratory force >20 cmH$_2$O

Why should nutrition be optimised prior to extubating the chronically ventilated?

There are two main reasons

- Nutritional state affects respiratory muscle strength and fatigability
- Excess reliance on glucose as the major source of carbohydrate leads to increased CO_2 production. This may lead to increased ventilator demands, and so failure to wean

▼

Briefly mention some of the ventilation strategies used to wean from mechanical ventilation.

- *T-piece ventilation:* added to the end of the circuit, and can be used just prior to extubation. When used on its own, it is more successful in those who have been intubated for a short period of time only (a couple of days at the maximum)

- *T piece and CPAP:* one of the problems of intubation is that it abolishes the small amount of natural PEEP provided by the laryngeal complex. The use of CPAP adds to the PEEP, permitting the T-piece to be used for longer periods in those who require it. Thus, during weaning, the T-piece is left on during parts of the day, while mechanical ventilation is continued at night

- *Intermittent mandatory ventilation (IMV):* the ventilator provides a certain tidal volume at a specified rate. Between these mechanical breaths, the patient supplements with their own, spontaneous breaths. The mandatory rate is progressively reduced, while increasing the spontaneous breaths

- *Pressure support ventilation:* the patient breathes spontaneously, but each breath is augmented with a positive inspiratory pressure. This is progressively reduced until full extubation, or CPAP

FAT EMBOLISM SYNDROME

What is the aetiology of fat embolism syndrome?

Traumatic or non-traumatic critical illness may trigger the fat embolism syndrome.

- Long bone fractures: especially of the femur or tibia. More common with closed fractures, possibly since the higher intra-medullary pressure forces more fat molecules into the circulation
- Major burns
- Acute pancreatitis: possibly related to pancreatic lipase activity
- Diabetes mellitus
- Orthopaedic procedures, e.g. joint reconstruction
- Decompression sickness
- Cardio-pulmonary bypass

What is the pathophysiology of how fat embolism syndrome develops?

There are two main theories

- *Mechanical theory:* this states that the fat droplets gain access to the circulation from the damaged vasculature at the site of the fracture. They are carried to the pulmonary vascular bed where they enter the systemic circulation through arterio-venous shunts. Impaction of these fat emboli in terminal systemic vascular beds produces local ischaemia and tissue injury. This does not explain the non-traumatic cases of this syndrome

- *Biochemical theory:* this explains the syndrome in terms of the release and activation of lipases by stress hormones such as steroids and catecholamines. Lipase hydolyses circulating platelet-bound lipids into free fatty acids (FFA) and glycerol. These FFAs induce pulmonary damage and increase capillary permeability. Platelet activation also releases 5 hydroxy-tryptamine, stimulating bronchospasm and vasospasm

▼

What are the clinical features of fat embolism syndrome and how do they relate to the pathophysiology?

There are a number of clinical features suggesting the syndrome has started. Ninety percent of these establish themselves within 3 days of the onset of the trigger.

Classically, there is the triad of cerebral signs, respiratory insufficiency and a petechial rash.

- *Cerebral features:* usually the earliest and most common clinical sign, occurring in up to 90% of those with the syndrome. Mainly presents as encephalopathy or as a distinct peripheral deficit such as hemiparesis. It is believed that this is due to
  - Microvessel embolisation of fat and platelet aggregates
  - Activated lipase damaging the lipid–rich cerebral matter
- *Respiratory insufficiency:* seen as tachypnoea and cyanosis 2–3 days following the initial insult. This is due to
  - Pulmonary vascular occlusion by lipid emboli leading to V/Q mismatch and increased shunt
  - Pneumonitis due to mediator release leading to increased capillary permeability and microatelectasis. This can lead to pulmonary oedema progressing to the syndrome of acute lung injury or ARDS
  - Superadded pneumonia
- *Petechial rash:* usually seen within 36 h as a purpura distributed in the area of the chest, axilla, mouth and conjunctiva. Arises as a result of
  - Direct embolisation to cutaneous vessels
  - Following thrombocytopenia due to platelet consumption as part of overall pathophysiology

There are a number of less common clinical features that may be seen

- Pyrexia of >38°C
- Tachycardia: may be a sign of right ventricular strain

- Retinopathy: following retinal artery embolisation
- Renal impairment: with oliguria, lipiduria and haematuria

Which of these features is pathognomic?

In the right clinical setting, the presence of a petechial rash is pathognomic of the fat embolisation syndrome.

What is the role of further investigations in making the diagnosis of fat embolism syndrome?

Given the importance of clinical signs in making the diagnosis of this condition, further investigations have a limited role. They are mainly used in assessing the severity of the condition, and mapping out organ system involvement when planning a management strategy.

- *Arterial blood gas analysis:* showing a V/Q mismatch which may be severe enough to produce a type I respiratory failure
- *Full blood count*
  - Decreased Hb: from trauma
  - Decreased platelet count
  - Elevated ESR
- *Clotting screen*
  - Increased fibrin-degradation products
  - Increased APTT
  - Increased TT
- *Serum electrolytes*
  - Assesses renal function
  - Reduced serum calcium: due to chelation by circulating lipids
- *Urine:* showing lipiduria
- *Sputum:* shows lipid-laden macrophages, and stains for lipid (e.g. by oil red-O)
- *Chest radiograph:* showing pulmonary infiltrates (described as a 'snow-storm' appearance) or infection

- *ECG:* showing tachycardia and right ventricular strain (flipped-T waves in the anterior leads)

How is fat embolism syndrome managed?

Management lies, in the main, with supportive measures for the affected organ systems, and the prevention of complications such as renal failure, pulmonary oedema and ARDS.

A number of specific treatments can also be used in an attempt to halt the progression, but these are unproven.

Supportive measures

- *Respiratory support:* with oxygenation. Can be administered as CPAP, or with mechanical ventilation if there are signs of ARDS
- *Fluid and electrolyte balance:* if too dry, there will be worsening renal function and acidosis, if overloaded, then there is exacerbation of pulmonary oedema
- *General measures:* such as DVT prophylaxis, nutritional support, control of sepsis etc

Specific therapies: these are unproven, but are based on an understanding of the pathophysiology.

- *i.v. ethanol:* reduces lipase activity
- *Dextran 40:* used to reduce platelet and red cell aggregation, and expand the plasma – but can worsen renal dysfunction
- *Heparin:* increases lipase activity, which can reduce circulating lipids. But it increases lipase-induced tissue injury and exacerbates haemorrhage in the trauma patient
- *Albumin solution:* binds to FFA. But if it leaks through permeable capillaries in the lung, can make pulmonary oedema worse

Can fat embolism syndrome be prevented?

Yes, a number of prophylactic measures may be used to prevent progression to the syndrome

- *Steroids:* there is some evidence that early use of methylprednisolone is beneficial

- *Early oxygen therapy:* CPAP can be used to reduce V/Q deficit by limiting atelectasis
- *Expedient fracture reduction and immobilisation:* limits the lipid load onto the circulation

What is the prognosis once fat embolism syndrome has established itself?

The mortality rate remains at 10–15%, but some of this is reflected in mortality from the underlying cause.

FLAIL CHEST

F

What are the defining features of a flail chest injury?

A flail chest occurs when there are three or more ribs fractured at two or more places on the rib shaft. This gives rise to an area of the chest wall that has lost bony continuity with the rest of the rib cage and has the potential to move autonomously during the respiratory cycle.

How much blood may be lost from a single rib fracture?

A rib fracture may be associated with the loss of 150 ml of blood.

What are the implications of finding a flail segment?

- It is a severity marker for the mechanism of injury: it takes a lot of kinetic injury to fracture several ribs at once owing to their elastic properties
- Thus, it may often occur with other thoracic injuries, such as pulmonary contusion, haemo/pneumothorax, blunt cardiac trauma or diaphragmatic rupture
- If severe enough, flail chest injuries may lead to respiratory failure in the absence of other associated thoracic injuries
- Later complications may arise, such as pneumonia and septicaemia. These are complications of retained secretions and atelectasis that occur following this injury

What are the pathophysiological changes to the respiratory system that can occur with flail chest injury?

Respiratory sequelae are

- The flail segment may exhibit paradoxical motion during the respiratory cycle, i.e. it moves inwards during inspiration. This is because it is drawn in by the increasing negativity of the intrapleural pressure, reducing the tidal volume

- Pain from the injury also reduces the tidal volume
- Reduced tidal volumes together with an inefficient cough mechanism leads to retention of secretions
- The resulting atelectasis causes V/Q mismatching that can lead to type I respiratory failure
- Ventilatory (type II) respiratory failure may also occur following the loss of the normal chest wall mechanical apparatus
- Underlying pulmonary contusion can exacerbate all of these effects

What are the principles of management of flail chest injury?

This injury must be managed in the context of the ATLS system

- Management of the flail segment itself
- Identification of injuries to the underlying thoracic organs
- Prevention of secondary complications such as atelectasis and pneumonia

The vast majority of patients may be conservatively managed and surgical intervention in the form of chest wall fixation is rarely required

- Humidified oxygen
- Adequate analgesia for pain relief, helping to improve respiratory physiology and permitting effective physiotherapy
- Intubation and mechanical ventilation in cases of worsening fatigue and respiratory failure
- Minitracheostomy, to help in the clearance of secretions may help to avert mechanical ventilation in the progressively decompensating patient

How may pain relief be achieved in these cases?

Analgesia, such as paracetamol, anti-inflammatory agents or opiates may be given enterally or parenterally. A commonly used parenteral route is thoracic epidural anaesthesia, with the level of the block extending to T4.

What is a 'sucking' chest wound, and how may it be immediately managed in the emergency setting?

A sucking chest wound occurs when the diameter of an open chest wall defect is greater than 2/3 the diameter of the trachea. Consequently, on inspiration, air preferentially enters the chest cavity directly through the open wound, not escaping on expiration. It therefore leads to a rapidly developing tension pneumothorax. In the emergency setting, it is managed by applying an occlusive dressing that is covered on three sides. This acts as a flutter-valve, preventing air entering on inspiration, and permitting air to escape on expiration.

FLUID THERAPY

How do you assess clinically the state of hydration?

- Examining the fluid chart for the input/output balance
- Examining the patient specifically looking for the state of the tissues
  - Skin turgor
  - Dry mouth
  - Sunken eyes
- Concentrated urine in the catheter
- Possible tachycardia and hypotension
- Measure the central venous pressure (CVP), and determine the response to a fluid challenge. If there is 'underfilling', the CVP will not increase in response to the challenge

What are the main fluid compartments of the body, and what are their volumes?

The fluid compartments are

- *Intracellular compartment:* 28 l
- *Extracellular compartment:* 14 l
  - Plasma: 3 l
  - Interstitium: 10 l
  - Transcellular: 1 l

Therefore the total body water is 42 l, which makes up ~60% of the body weight of a 70 kg male and 55–60% for females.

How can the percentage fall of the extracellular fluid volume be calculated?

In the case of loss of extracellular fluid (ECF), the concentration of the plasma albumin increases depending on the amount of water lost during dehydration. The resulting rise in

▼

the albumin concentration can be used to calculate the % fall in the ECF volume.

$$\% \text{ fall in the ECF volume} = \left(1 - \frac{A1}{A2}\right) \times 100$$

where $A1$ = initial albumin concentration; $A2$ = albumin concentration following loss of volume.

How can the percentage fall in the plasma volume be calculated?

In situations of loss of plasma, there is a loss of plasma protein, but not of blood. Thus, the haematocrit increases in proportion to the volume of plasma lost. Measurements of the haematocrit are therefore useful in calculating the % fall in the plasma volume.

$$\% \text{ fall in the plasma volume}$$
$$= 100 \left[1 - \left(\frac{HCT1}{100 - HCT1} \times \frac{100 - HCT2}{HCT2}\right)\right]$$

where $HCT1$ = initial haematocrit; $HCT2$ = haematocrit after plasma loss.

What is the basal water requirement for an adult?

30–40 ml/kg/day.

What is the purpose of fluid therapy?

- To satisfy part or the entire basal requirement of water
- To satisfy part or the entire basal requirement of electrolytes
- To replace fluid and electrolytes lost beyond the basal requirements
- To support the arterial pressure in cases of shock by increasing the plasma volume and improving tissue perfusion
- If given as blood, to increase the oxygen carrying capacity of the blood

F

What types of fluids are available?

Fluids may be given as

- *Colloids:* these may be naturally occurring or synthetic, being composed of large molecules generally with a molecular weight of >30,000. They confine themselves to the plasma, exerting an osmotic pressure (unless there is injury to capillary integrity, when they can leak into the interstitium)

- *Crystalloids:* these solutions are able to more easily pass between compartments. In the case of 5% dextrose, once the dextrose is metabolised, the remaining water distributes itself in the total body water

By which routes may fluids be administered?

- Enteral
- i.v.
- Subcutaneous: particularly if i.v. access is difficult
- Intraosseous: using a metal cannula into the medullary cavity of the tibia (beneath the tibial tuberosity), or into the iliac crest

When is the intraosseous route used?

Intraosseous fluid administration is reserved for children under the age of 6 years when conventional access is not possible.

Would you use crystalloids or colloids in the emergency setting?

Either may be used but this is controversial. Both are able to provide plasma volume expansion in the support of the arterial pressure during blood loss. Crystalloids, however have no oxygen carrying capacity unlike blood (a colloid). This is likely to be required in cases of severe blood loss when tissue oxygenation is diminished further by loss of red cells. Also, because of the volume of distribution of crystalloid, more of it is required than colloid to provide a comparable increase in the plasma volume.

▼

What is the composition of Hartmann's solution and how does it compare to normal (0.9%) saline?

Hartmann's solution is composed of

- Sodium: 131 mmol/l
- Potassium: 5 mmol/l
- Chloride: 111 mmol/l
- Bicarbonate: 29 mmol/l (provided as lactate, which is metabolised to bicarbonate)
- It has an osmolality of 280 mOsm/l

Normal (0.9%) saline contains only sodium and chloride at a concentration of 150 mmol/l. It is also iso-osmolar with plasma with an osmolality of 300 mOsm/l (i.e. 150 + 150).

What types of colloid are available, and what are the basic characteristics of each?

The colloids available are

- *Blood*
- *Human albumin solution* (4.5 or 20%): obtained by fractionation of plasma, having a molecular weight of 69,000. Not only provides plasma expansion, but acts as a carrier molecule and buffer. Plasma half-life is measured in days (~10 days or more)
- *Dextrans* (40 or 70 depending on the molecular weight): artificial colloids composed of branched polysaccharide. The plasma half-life is in the order of 12 h. Dextran 70 reduces platelet adhesion, and interferes with blood cross matching. Also carries a risk of anaphylaxis
- *Gelatins:* formed from the hydrolysis of bovine collagen. Have a short plasma half-life – in the order of 2–4 h, being rapidly excreted by the kidneys. There are three main types
  - Succinylated gelatins, e.g. Gelofusin
  - Urea cross-linked gelatins, e.g. Haemaccel
  - Oxypolygelatins

They also have a long shelf life (3 years).

- *Starches:* examples are 6% hetastarch (Hespan, Elo-HAES), or pentastarch. These consist of chains of glucose molecules. The average molecular weight is 70,000, but some molecules in the mixture are much larger. Therefore, can be useful in cases of capillary leakage when smaller colloids may worsen interstitial oedema. Also, the dose of Hetastarch must be limited to 1500 ml/day due to the risk of coagulopathy. The plasma half-life is ~24 h

What are the precautions with using colloids?

- *Potential risk of disease transmission:* with blood and blood products

- *Coagulopathy:* Dextran 70, gelatins, and high molecular weight starches interfere with platelet adhesion and von Willebrand factor

- *Interaction with blood transfusion:* the calcium content of Haemaccel can cause blood to clot if infused into the same cannula

- *Immunological reactions:* other than blood, Dextran 70, and gelatins may cause pruritis or anaphylaxis. May also occur with starches, but much more rarely

- *Risk of worsening oedema:* if loss of capillary integrity causes the colloid to leak into the interstitial compartment

HAEMORRHAGIC SHOCK

What is the definition of shock?

This is a syndrome of inadequacy of tissue perfusion to meet the metabolic demands of the body and is associated with the features of a sympathoadrenal and neuroendocrine response.

What types of shock are there?

The types of shock may be classified as

- Hypovolaemic
- Cardiogenic
- With reduced systemic vascular resistance
  - Septic shock: associated with gram negative organisms
  - Anaphylactic shock: associated with a type I hypersensitivity reaction
  - Neurogenic shock: loss of sympathetic outflow following spinal cord injury
- With obstruction to blood flow
  - Massive pulmonary embolism
  - Cardiac tamponade

Give some causes of hypovolaemic shock.

- Haemorrhage: which may be occult
- Burns: following the loss of the protective epidermis
- Dehydration:
  - Inadequate intake
  - Loss from the gut, e.g. vomiting, diarrhoea
  - Renal losses: diuretic abuse, osmotic diuresis of diabetic ketoacidosis, Addisonian crisis

Give some common causes of acute occult bleeding that can give rise to hypovolaemic shock.

- Closed fractures of the femur or pelvis
- Blunt chest trauma: injuring the heart, intercostal, internal thoracic or great vessels

- Blunt abdominal injury with bleeding from the liver or splenic bed
- Retroperitoneal bleed: may occur with ruptured aneurysms
- Obstetric haemorrhage: abruptio placenta, placenta accreta, retained products
- Post-operative exsanguination into a body cavity

How may the severity of blood loss be classified?

There are four classes depending on the volume lost
- Class I: <500 ml (<10% of circulating volume)
- Class II: 500–1000 ml (10–20% of circulating volume)
- Class III: 1000–2000 ml (20–40%)
- Class IV: >2000 ml (>40%)

How much blood may be lost from fractures of the pelvis, femur and tibia?

- Pelvic fractures, 1–3 l
- Femoral fractures, 1–2 l
- Tibial fractures, 0.5–1 l

Outline the cardiovascular response to blood loss.

The stimulus to the various responses to hypovolaemia comes from a reduction of the venous return (preload) giving rise to a fall in the cardiac output and arterial pressure, by the Frank–Starling mechanism.

- The baroreceptor reflex stimulates sympathetic activity, leading to a compensatory tachycardia, increased stroke volume with peripheral vaso- and venoconstriction
- This has the effect of increasing the cardiac output
- Pain and injury also stimulates catecholamine release from the adrenal medulla – particularly norepinephrine, which increases the peripheral vascular resistance
- Release of corticosteroids from the adrenal cortex stimulates salt and water retention and stimulates the systemic stress response

- In the medium term, the reduction in the circulating volume and increased sympathetic activity stimulates the release of renin from the macula densa of the juxta-glomerular apparatus of the kidney. This leads to the renin–angiotensin–aldosterone cascade. There is salt and water retention, helping to restore the circulating volume over the next few hours
- Reduction of renal perfusion stimulates erythropoetin production, and thus erythropoesis

What are the clinical features of haemorrhagic shock?

Clinical features depend on the volume of blood loss, and the degree of compensation. Features include

- Tachycardia
- Initial normal blood pressure with a narrowed pulse pressure
- Cool peripheries: a sign of redistribution of blood to more important organ systems
- Reduced CVP, with a transient, unsustained rise following fluid challenge
- Reduced urine output
- Confusion: due to reduced cerebral perfusion

What features are seen as the patient decompensates?

- Reduction of the level of consciousness
- Falling arterial pressure
- Worsening lactic acidosis: consequent upon a sustained poor peripheral perfusion stimulating anaerobic metabolism
- Bradycardia

Why do decompensating patients often become bradycardic?

Bradycardia may arise from a number of factors

- Stimulation of the 'depressor reflex': deformation of the ventricular wall occurring as a result of poor ventricular filling leads to activation of vagal C-fibre afferents in the myocardium. This leads to increased vagal activity, manifesting as bradycardia associated with blood loss. It is thought that this reflex has the protective effect of reducing the myocardial oxygen demand when the coronary perfusion is poor, at the expense of causing decompensation

- Myocardial activity may be impaired by persisting ischaemia

Define the haematocrit (packed cell volume). What is the normal level?

This is the proportion of the total blood volume that consists of the red cells. It may be expressed as a percentage or a fraction of the blood volume. It is 0.4–0.54 in males, and 0.37–0.47 in females.

What factors determine the haematocrit?

This is determined by

- Changes in the total red cell volume: e.g. due to blood loss
- Changes in the plasma volume: e.g. losses of water, or plasma expansion that occurs in pregnancy or fluid overload
- Sex of the individual – being greater in men
- Venous or arterial blood: The volume of red cells in venous blood is slightly higher than in arterial blood due to entry of water with chloride ions during the chloride shift that occurs with CO_2-carriage. Therefore, the packed cell volume in venous blood is higher

What are the consequences of a change in the haematocrit?

The implications are

- Alterations in the oxygen-carrying capacity of the blood
- Changes in the viscosity of the blood, which affect the rate and pattern of blood flow in the vascular tree

▼

How can the blood volume be calculated from the plasma volume?

$$\text{Blood volume} = \text{plasma volume} \times \frac{100}{100 - \text{haematocrit}}$$

What is the basic management of blood loss?

The basic management involves

- Gaining adequate vascular access. The Hagen–Poiseuille equation states that fluid flow through a tube is proportional to the fourth power of the radius of the tube, and inversely proportional to its length. Thus, the most immediately useful form of access is a wide-bore peripheral cannula, not a central line

- Supporting the arterial pressure with a fluid infusion to improve the venous return. Pneumatic anti-shock trousers have also been used to improve the venous return

- Crystalloids and colloids may help to increase the blood pressure, and therefore improve peripheral organ perfusion. However, they do not improve the oxygen carrying capacity of the blood – only a blood transfusion may do this. Therefore, a transfusion is organised in more severe cases of blood loss

- The success of resuscitation can be assessed with the aid of a urinary catheter to measure the urine output, and a central line to assess cardiac filling

- If there is an open site of bleeding, it may be controlled by digital pressure

- Ultimately, following initial recitation and stabilisation, surgical intervention may be required to stem further loss of blood, e.g. laparotomy, thoracotomy, fracture immobilisation

- Note that, in the case of trauma, all of this should be performed in the context of the ABCD of the primary survey during C-spine control

HEAD INJURY I – PHYSIOLOGY

What is the volume of the cerebrospinal fluid (CSF)?
140–150 ml.

Where is CSF produced, and at what rate?
70% of CSF is produced by the choroid plexus of the lateral, third and fourth ventricles. 30% comes directly from the vessels lining the ventricular walls. It is produced at a rate of 0.35 ml/min, or ~500 ml/day.

Briefly describe the circulation of CSF.
From the lateral ventricle, the CSF flows into the third ventricle through the interventricular foramen of Monro. From here it enters into the fourth ventricle through the aqueduct of Sylvius. Some continue down into the central canal of the spinal cord, but the majority flow into the sub-arachnoid space of the spinal cord via the central foramen of Magendie, or the two lateral foramina of Luschka. After going around the spinal cord, it enters the cranial cavity through the foramen magnum, and flows around the brain within the sub-arachnoid space.

What are the arachnoid villi composed of?
The arachnoid villi are formed from a fusion of arachnoid membrane and the endothelium of the dural venous sinus that it has bulged into.

Where is the CSF finally absorbed?
80% of CSF is absorbed at the arachnoid villi, and 20% is absorbed at the spinal nerve roots.

What structures form the blood–brain barrier (BBB)?
The BBB, which is a histological and physiological boundary between the blood and the CSF, is formed from two types of special anatomical arrangement

- Tight junctions in-between the endothelial cells of the cerebral capillaries

▼

- Astrocytic foot processes applied to the basal membranes of the cerebral capillaries

What substances can pass through the BBB?

The BBB is permeable to lipids, lipid soluble molecules (such as opiates and general anaesthetics), respiratory gases and glucose. Chronically, it is also permeable to protons (H^+).

Which parts of the brain lie outside of the BBB?

Three main areas lie outside of the BBB

- The posterior lobe of the pituitary gland (neurohypophysis): which produces vasopressin and oxytocin
- Circumventricular organs around the 3rd and 4th ventricles: such as the supraoptic crest, the area postrema and tuber cinerium
- The median eminence of the hypothalamus

Which pathologies can affect the integrity of the BBB?

BBB integrity is lost by infection, tumours, trauma, and ischaemia.

What is the cerebral blood flow?

50 ml/100 g of tissue. The total flow is ~750 ml/min, or ~15% of the cardiac output.

How does cerebral blood flow vary with the arterial pressure?

Between systolic pressures of 50–150 mmHg, the cerebral blood flow remains constant owing to local autoregulation of flow.

What is the mechanism of autoregulation?

There are two main factors that allow the cerebral blood flow to remain constant despite variations in the driving pressure:

- *Myogenic response of the arteriolar smooth muscle cells:* an increase in the wall tension caused by a rise in the mean arterial pressure stimulates a reactive contraction of the cells. This increases the vascular resistance, keeping the flow constant

- *Vasodilator 'washout':* if blood flow is momentarily increased by a sudden rise in arterial pressure, locally-produced vasodilator substances are washed out, leading to increased vascular resistance, and so a return of flow back to the normal

What other factors regulate the cerebral blood flow?

Blood flow is affected by

- *Carbon dioxide:* hypercarbia increases the cerebral blood flow through an increased $[H^+]$. Conversely, hypocarbia leads to cerebral vasoconstriction

- *Hypoxia:* produces vasodilatation (less pronounced and more delayed in comparison to that in response to hypercarbia)

- *Sympathetic innervation of cerebral vessels:* this has a minor effect on the cerebral flow

Define the cerebral perfusion pressure.

The cerebral perfusion pressure is defined as the difference between mean arterial pressure and intracranial pressure (Mean arterial pressure − intracranial pressure).

It must remain above ~70 mmHg for the brain tissue to be adequately perfused.

What is the Cushing reflex?

This is mixed vagal and sympathetic stimulation that occurs in response to an elevated intracranial pressure. It leads to hypertension, which ensures an adequate cerebral perfusion pressure. There is also a resultant bradycardia.

HEAD INJURY II – PATHOPHYSIOLOGY

What does the Monro–Kellie doctrine state?

This states that the cranial cavity can be considered to be a rigid sphere, filled to capacity with non-compressible contents – brain, blood and CSF. Consequently, an increase of one of these contents necessarily causes a displacement of the others to a varying degree.

Draw a graph showing the relationship of the intracranial pressure (ICP) to the intracranial volume. What does this show?

This shows the changing nature of the compliance of the intracranial contents with increases in the ICP. Initially, due to a higher intracranial compliance, a small rise in the volume leads to little rise in the ICP. At a higher volume, there is an exponential rise in the ICP owing to the contents becoming 'stiffer' due to volume overload. The volume at which this ICP decompensation occurs differs among individuals.

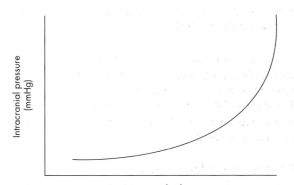

Intracranial volume

The relationship between the
intracranial volume & intracranial pressure

Adapted from journal article, "Applied physiology of the CNS" by MA Glasby & LM Myles in Sugery (2000) 18(9): iii–vi page iv, Diagram 1.

Give some basic causes of a raised ICP.

- Increase of CSF: hydrocephalus
- Increase of blood: intracranial bleeding – subdural, extradural, subarachnoid, and intracerebral
- Increase of brain: tumours, cerebral oedema, benign intracranial hypertension

What are the signs and symptoms of a raised ICP?

The four cardinal signs and symptoms of a raised ICP are

- *Headache:* often worse in the morning
- *Nausea and vomiting:* worse in the morning
- *Reduced level of consciousness:* may manifest as simple drowsiness. This is an important sign, since its significance may be missed
- *Papilloedema:* a definitive sign of raised ICP, as the pressure is transmitted along the subarachnoid space of the optic nerve
- In the infant (below 18 months) there may be a tense anterior fontanelle

What is the most important and life-threatening complication of raised ICP?

The most significant complication is cerebral herniation which can lead to rapid onset of coma, respiratory failure, and death.

What varieties of brain herniation are there, and how may they manifest themselves?

There are three types of brain herniation

- *Subfalcine:* where the cingulate gyrus herniates beneath the falx cerebri
- *Foramen magnum herniation:* leading to displacement of the medulla and the cerebellar tonsils. Compression of the respiratory centre leads to respiratory depression
- *Transtentorial:* the uncus of the temporal lobe passes through the tentorial hiatus

▼

Herniation can lead to a number of effects

- With transtentorial herniation, can lead to ipsilateral compression of the oculomotor nerve (CN III) and pyramidal tract running in the midbrain. This is clinically manifest as an ipsilateral dilated pupil and a contralateral hemiparesis

- Displacement of the posterior cerebral artery may produce visual field defects with transtentorial herniation

- Pressure on the brainstem stimulates Cheyne–Stokes respiration and the Cushing reflex

- Exponential rise in the ICP as flow of the CSF is suddenly occluded by the herniated brain

Name a 'false localising sign' – why does this occur?

The classical false localising sign is an abducent (CN VI) nerve palsy, with an inability to abduct the eye. This falsely points to the abducent motor nucleus as being the site of the lesion. In reality it results from herniation producing kinking of the sixth nerve as it runs a long intracranial course.

HEAD INJURY III – PRINCIPLES OF MANAGEMENT

What is the incidence of death from a head injury in the UK?

In the UK death from head injuries account for 9 deaths per 100,000 population per year.

Which age range is most at risk?

Most of the deaths occur in those aged between 5–35 years. Head injury accounts for 15–20% of deaths in this group.

What is the risk of an intracranial bleed in the patient with a minor head injury without a fracture or amnesia?

If the patient is orientated then the risk is said to be 1 in 6000. If disorientated, then the risk is 1 in 120.

What is the principle of management of the patient with a minor head injury?

By definition, the GCS is 14–15. The principles of management revolve around two key questions

- Does the patient require any form of imaging?
- Does the patient require admission for observation?

Those who are conscious with no evidence of a fracture may be discharged into the care of a responsible adult with written advice. Others are admitted for a period of observation (at least 4 h).

When would you perform a CT scan?

- Persisting neurological signs following resuscitation
- Persisting headache or vomiting
- Falling level of consciousness

▼

- Suspicion of a base of skull fracture: CSF oto-/rhinorrhoea, or subconjunctival haemorrhage with no posterior limit, periorbital haematoma, Battle's sign
- Suspected penetrating injury

Briefly outline a strategy for the management of the severely head injured patient.

Management involves

- Discussion with the local neurosurgical unit at an early opportunity
- Following an assessment of the severity of the primary injury, secondary brain injury must be prevented
- The patient may require intubation and ventilation to help control the $PaCO_2$ and hence the intracranial pressure. If the PaO_2 is >12 kPa, and the $PaCO_2$ <6 kPa with an FiO_2 of 0.4, then the patient may not require intubation.
- Other than controlling the ventilation, there are a number of other methods of reducing the intracranial pressure (*see* below)
- The mean arterial pressure must be maintained above 90 mmHg to help maintain the cerebral perfusion pressure above 65 mmHg
- If there is an intracranial haematoma causing a mass effect, then emergency surgical evacuation is required
- The intracranial pressure may be monitored using a probe or external ventricular drain. This also permits the calculation of the cerebral perfusion pressure
- Hyperthermia may occur due to hypothalamic dysfunction or infection. This can be managed with a cooling blanket
- Hyponatraemia may occur due to overhydration, the stress response to trauma with Na/water retention, or due to the syndrome of inappropriate ADH. This has to be managed by careful fluid and electrolyte balance, since hyponatraemia may lead to further neurological impairment and cerebral oedema

Why should the ICP be controlled?
What techniques are available?

There are two main reasons why the ICP should be controlled

- A high ICP can lead to cerebral herniation
- A high ICP causes a reduction of the cerebral perfusion pressure (since the cerebral perfusion pressure = mean arterial pressure − ICP)

There are a number of techniques used to reduce the ICP

- Controlled ventilation, keeping the $PaCO_2$ between 4–4.5 kPa. This controls the degree of intracranial vasodilatation
- Fluid restriction, which prevents cerebral oedema
- Diuretics, e.g. mannitol or furosemide. Mannitol is an osmotic diuretic given at a dose of 0.5–1.0 g/kg over 20 min. It can be used to 'buy time' while preparing for surgery
- Direct tapping off the CSF from a ventricular catheter
- Tilting the end of the bed 20 degrees
- Barbiturates, e.g. thiopentone if the ICP is resistant to the above measures
- Note that steroids are helpful in reducing the swelling around cerebral tumours, but not in situations of trauma

What are the other complications of a severe head injury?

- Shorter term:
  - *Meningitis and brain abscess:* where there has been an open communication
- Longer term:
  - *Epilepsy:* especially common in the situation of a depressed fracture, intracranial haematoma or prolonged amnesia
  - *Hydrocephalus:* caused by obstruction from an intraventricular haemorrhage

- *Chronic subdural haematoma:* may cause symptoms from a chronic elevation of the ICP, and managed by surgical evacuation
- *Cognitive symptoms:* e.g. post traumatic amnesia and post concussion symptoms such as persisting headaches, dizziness and poor concentration

INOTROPES AND CIRCULATORY SUPPORT

In which ways may the failing cardiovascular system be supported?

The cardiovascular system may need support if there is a fall in the cardiac index to below $2.2 l/min/m^2$, or in the situation of septic shock when peripheral circulatory failure results in a fall in the systemic vascular resistance (SVR) and arterial pressure. It may be supported by the following means

- Inotropic agents
- Vasoconstrictors
- Vasodilators
- Cardiac pacing to provide chronotropic support
- Mechanical circulatory support
  - Intra-aortic balloon pump counterpulsation
  - Ventricular assist devices

Give some examples of commonly used drugs for this purpose.

Examples include

- *Adrenergic agonists:* epinephrine, norepinephrine, isoprenaline

- *Dopaminergic agents (with some adrenergic activity):* dopamine, dobutamine, dopexamine

- *Phosphodiesterase inhibitors:* milrinone, enoximone

- *Calcium chloride,* producing a transient inotropic effect

Elaborate on the mechanism of action of the phosphodiesterase inhibitors.

The phosphodiesterase inhibitors act by inhibiting the degradation of intracellular cyclic AMP. This causes an increase in the intracellular concentration of calcium ions, leading to enhanced contractility

What is their effect on cardiovascular function?

These agents improve cardiac output by two important means

- Reduction of systemic and pulmonary vascular resistance leads to afterload reduction. Thus, particularly useful in the situation of cardiogenic shock associated with a high systemic vascular resistance. Also useful in cases of right ventricular dysfunction with pulmonary hypertension
- There is a moderate direct positive inotropic effect
- There is a reduction in the myocardial oxygen demand due to a lowering of filling pressures

Draw a diagram comparing the effects of the different inotropes on adrenergic receptors.

Drug	α_1	β_1	β_2	DA_1	Dose (μg/kg/min)
Dopamine					
Low dose				+++	1–4
Medium dose		+	+	+++	5–10
High dose	+	+	+	+++	>10

Comments
Dose-dependent effects. Increased splanchnic/renal blood flow and diuretic effect at low doses, but no evidence for renal protective activity. May inhibit gastric emptying

Dopexamine	0	0	+++	++	0.5–6

Comments
Inodilator licensed for treatment of heart failure following cardiac surgery. Increases hepatosplanchnic blood flow, and may ameliorate gut ischaemia in SIRS

Dobutamine	0	+++	++	0	2.5–10

Comments
Inodilator, useful in low output/high systemic vascular resistance (SVR) states such as cardiogenic shock.
Unlikely to be of benefit in the hypotension associated with sepsis/SIRS

Salbutamol	0	+	+++	0	0.1–1

Comments
Useful in treatment of acute severe asthma

Continued overleaf

Drug	α_1	β_1	β_2	DA_1	Dose (μg/kg/min)
Epinephrine	+ to +++	+++	++	0	0.01–0.2

Comments
Useful first-line inotrope. High β-adrenoceptor activity, increasing cardiac output. Vasodilatation may be seen at low doses, vasoconstriction at higher doses

Norepinephrine	+++	+	0	0	0.01–0.2

Comments
Inoconstrictor. Very useful in high output/low SVR states such as severe SIRS/sepsis. Inotropic effect via myocardial α-receptors and β-activity. May cause reflex bradycardia. Risk of peripheral and splanchnic ischaemia

Isoprenaline	0	+++	+++	0	0.01–0.2

Comments
Potent β-agonist, hence risk of tachydysrhythmias. Generally reserved for emergency treatment of bradydysrhythmias and AV block prior to pacing. Now replaced by salbutamol in the management of acute severe asthma

Phenylephrine	+++	0	0	0	0.2–1

Comments
Pure vasoconstrictor. Useful alternative to norepinephrine (e.g. if arrhythmias are a problem)

Before inotropes are commenced, what safeguards must be in place?

Prior to the use of inotropes, adequate cardiovascular monitoring should be in place – the minimum being the presence of continuous ECG monitoring, pulse oximetry, urinary catheter and a central (right atrial) catheter.

What are the effects of dopamine on the circulation?

In low doses (<5 μg/kg/min) dopamine acts on dopaminergic receptors. At a higher dose (>15 μg/kg/min) it acts on β receptors. At this high dose, and faster infusion rates, it also acts on α receptors. Thus at low doses it causes renal and mesenteric vasodilatation, causing diuresis and natriuresis. However, evidence suggests that some of the improved urine output is due to a direct inotropic effect. At higher doses causes vasoconstriction and tachyarrhythmias.

What are the indications for the use of norepinephrine?

Norepinephrine, having mainly α effects, is a potent vasoconstrictor that is useful in supporting the arterial pressure in cases of septic shock. The resulting vasoconstriction leads to reduced peripheral perfusion at higher doses despite improved arterial pressure. It can also be used with the phosphodiesterase inhibitors, so the patient benefits from increased ejection fraction, without excessive vasodilatation.

What are the effects of epinephrine on the circulation?

At low doses, the β effects predominate. At higher doses, the α effects predominate. Thus, at low doses it increases the cardiac output and reduces the SVR. At higher doses, there is an increase in the afterload and arterial pressure due to increases in the SVR. Although providing increased coronary blood flow, it also can increase the myocardial oxygen demand. It also causes lactic acidosis, even at low doses.

What about dobutamine?

Having strong β-1 effects, has both inotropic and chronotropic effects, increasing the cardiac output. Also reduces the systemic vascular resistance (β-2 stimulation), potentially leading to reduced blood pressure. It is useful in situations where the cardiac output is low with increased SVR.

What are the general problems associated with the use of inotropes?

Some of the problems of inotropic agents are

- Tachyarrhythmias
- Bradycardia, e.g. norepinephrine
- Hypertension, e.g. epinephrine
- Hypotension, e.g. dobutamine, phosphodiesterase inhibitors
- Increased myocardial oxygen consumption and demand

INOTROPES AND CIRCULATORY SUPPORT

What can be done if the cardiac index is still poor despite maximum inotrope use?

In these situations, the circulation can be supported with the use of an intra-aortic balloon pump which can be inserted in the ITU setting.

How does an intra-aortic balloon pump work?

The basic principle involves mechanical assistance to the failing heart through afterload reduction and an improvement of the coronary blood flow. The device sits in the descending aorta and is connected to an external console that pumps helium in and out of the balloon in phase with the ECG. The balloon expands in diastole, causing an increase in the coronary perfusion pressure. By deflating just before the onset of systole, it leads to afterload reduction, reducing impedance to left ventricular ejection and reduced myocardial workload.

How and where is intra-aortic balloon inserted?

It may be inserted at the time of cardiac surgery or in the ITU through the femoral artery at the groin, using the Seldinger technique.

ITU ADMISSION CRITERIA

What are the levels of intensity of care of hospital patients?

Care of hospital patients may be divided into four levels

- *Level 0:* the ward environment meeting the needs of the patient
- *Level 1:* the ward patient requires the input of the critical care team for advice on optimisation of care
- *Level 2:* high dependency unit care – more detailed observation and intervention is required, often for a single failing organ system, or following major surgery
- *Level 3:* ITU care for the support and management of two or more failing systems or for advanced respiratory support

What is the purpose of the intensive care unit?

The intensive care unit provides advanced respiratory, cardiovascular and renal monitoring and support. It follows that conditions requiring support and monitoring must be thought reversible at the time of admission to the unit.

Give some criteria for admitting patients to the ITU.

- Advanced respiratory support is required, i.e. intubation and mechanical ventilation
- Two or more organs need to be supported
- The disease process is considered to be reversible
- The wishes of the patient are not breached

How does the cost of ITU care compare to ordinary ward care?

It has been estimated that ITU care is some 3–4 times more expensive than routine ward care.

What other departments must be found in the vicinity of the ITU?

- The operating rooms
- Imaging department
- Accident and Emergency
- Obstetric department

JUGULAR VENOUS PULSE (JVP)

Which of the jugular veins is used for examination of the JVP, and why?

The internal jugular vein. The lack of valves in this vessel, unlike in the external jugular, provides a single column of blood that is directly affected by events in the right heart and thoracic cavity.

What information may be obtained from an examination of the JVP?

Examining the height of the JVP provides a clinical measure of the CVP, which equates to the right atrial pressure. Therefore, it gives information on circulatory volume and right ventricular function. Observing the waveform of the JVP may give information about the patient's heart rhythm, as well as right heart function.

How may it be distinguished from the carotid pulse?

- There are two ('a' and 'v') venous pulsations to each carotid pulse
- The venous pulse is obliterated by light pressure at the root of the neck
- The height of the JVP varies with the respiratory cycle
- Abdominal compression causes a momentary rise in the JVP (hepato-jugular reflex)

Draw the normal JVP waveform, explaining how the differing wave deflections come about.

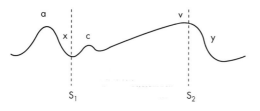

The Jugular venous pulse waveform in relation to the first (S_1) and second (S_2) heart sounds.

- *a* wave is due to atrial contraction
- *x* descent follows atrial relaxation
- *c* wave produced by bulging of the tricuspid valve into the atrium at the start of ventricular systole
- *v* wave occurs as a result of venous return to the atrium. It indicates the timing of ventricular systole, but is not caused by it
- *y* descent occurs at the opening of the tricuspid valve

What are the causes of an elevated JVP?

Some of the causes include

- Obstruction of flow into the right atrium: obstructed SVC, e.g. due to lung tumour, mediastinal mass or large goitre. There is a loss of the waveforms
- Disease at the level of the right atrio–ventricular junction: tricuspid valve stenosis or incompetence, right atrial myxoma (rare)
- Elevations of the intrathoracic pressure being transmitted to the right atrium, e.g. large pleural effusion, tension pneumothorax
- Over-filled right atrium: excess fluid administration, failing right ventricle
- Compressed right ventricle: tamponade, constrictive pericarditis

How does the waveform differ in cases of atrial fibrillation, complete heart block, tricuspid stenosis and incompetence?

- *Atrial fibrillation:* absent '*a*' wave. Timing with the carotid pulse shows that the impulses are 'irregularly irregular'
- *Complete heart block:* 'cannon' '*a*' wave due to discordant atrial and ventricular contractions leading to situations where the atrium occasionally contracts against a closed tricuspid valve, transmitting a large wave to the internal jugular

- *Tricuspid stenosis:* large '*a*' wave due to obstruction at the atrio-ventricular level and slow '*y*' descent due to slow atrial emptying
- *Tricuspid incompetence:* large '*v*' wave due to surging of right ventricular blood into the atrium through an incompetent valve during ventricular systole

Why does the height of the JVP vary with the respiratory cycle?

During inspiration, the intrathoracic pressure falls (becomes more negative) increasing the flow of blood back to the heart. Therefore, the JVP falls as the column of blood flows into the heart. During expiration, the rise in the intrathoracic pressure reduces the venous return to the heart, causing an elevation of the JVP.

What is Kussmaul's sign?

Kussmaul's sign is a paradoxical rise in the JVP on inspiration. It occurs in situations where the right atrium cannot accommodate the increase in its venous return caused by a fall in the intrathoracic pressure on inspiration, e.g. in right heart failure and constrictive pericarditis.

J

JUGULAR VENOUS PULSE

LACTIC ACIDOSIS

What are the defining features of lactic acidosis?

The important features are the presence of a metabolic acidosis (with a varying degree of respiratory compensation), and an elevated serum lactate. The serum lactate is normally <2 mmol/l, but with lactic acidosis may increase to >5 mmol/l.

How may the causes of lactic acidosis be classified?

The Cohen and Woods (1976) classification divides the causes thus

- *Type A:*
  - Results from poor tissue perfusion and cellular hypoxia with resulting anaerobic metabolism
  - Lactate is generated from pyruvate
  - Can be caused by any cause of shock – cardiogenic, hypovolaemic, septic or obstructive
- *Type B:*
  - As a complication of other diseases: liver disease, renal failure, diabetic ketoacidosis, malignancy, short-bowel syndrome
  - Also, inborn error of metabolism: e.g. pyruvate dehydrogenase deficiency
  - May also be drug-induced: paracetamol/salicylate overdose, metformin, epinephrine, alcohol intoxication

What are the essential findings on investigation?

The diagnostic features are an elevated serum lactate, and the presence of an increased-anion gap metabolic acidosis in the face of known predisposing factors.

What are the principles of management of lactic acidosis?

The most important aspect of management is

- The management of the predisposing factor, e.g. support of the cardiac output in order to improve the tissue perfusion

▼

- i.v. bicarbonate has been used to help correct severe acidosis. This is controversial
- Other agents have been used as an alternative to bicarbonate to correct the acidosis, but they have an unproven benefit

What are the precautions and potential problems associated with bicarbonate therapy?

Some considerations must be made when using bicarbonate to reverse metabolic acidosis

- Bicarbonate must be infused slowly: it comes as a hypertonic 8.4% solution, which can lead to alterations of myocardial contractility depending on the rate of infusion
- The dose of bicarbonate must be carefully titrated to the desired therapeutic end-point. This is because of the risk of an 'overshoot' metabolic alkalosis
- 'Overshoot' alkalosis also shifts the oxygen dissociation curve to the *left*, reducing oxygen delivery to the tissues
- Ventilation must be adequate to blow off the extra CO_2 generated consequent upon the use of bicarbonate to 'mop-up' excess protons (H^+). If not, a respiratory acidosis may ensue
- Intracellular acidosis may also be worsened by the use of bicarbonate: unlike protons, CO_2 readily diffuses across cell membranes. It follows that the extra CO_2 generated by bicarbonate therapy can diffuse into cells, and the BBB. This CO_2 then dissolves in the cytoplasm (and CSF), generating extra protons, worsening intracellular and intracerebral acidosis

L

LOW URINE OUTPUT STATE

What is the purpose of measuring the urine output in the post-operative patient?

Since the urine output is determined by the renal perfusion pressure, measurement provides a useful index of the cardiac output, and the ability to adequately oxygenate the peripheral tissues. It is also an indicator of renal tubular function, independent of the renal perfusion and cardiac output.

What is the minimum acceptable urine output in adults and children?

In adults, the minimum acceptable urine output is 0.5 ml/kg/h. In children, 1 ml/kg/h.

What factors determine the urine output?

- Adequate renal perfusion pressure – determined by the cardiac output and the arteriolar tone
- Normal renal tubular function
- Patent urinary tract distal to the kidneys

What are the common causes of post–operative oliguria?

- Physiological 'stress' response
- Poor renal perfusion
  - Dehydration/underfilling
  - Bleeding
  - Low cardiac output state
  - Vasodilatation, e.g. due to septic shock
- Renal tubular dysfunction: acute tubular necrosis and established renal failure
- Renal tract obstruction: e.g. due to stones, extrinsic compression, blocked urinary catheter
- Intra–abdominal hypertension (>20 mmHg): can occur with bowel obstruction or retroperitoneal collection, where there is compression of the renal parenchyma

L

Which pathologies may lead to a post-operative low cardiac output state?

A low cardiac output state post-operatively may be caused by

- Excess fluid administration, leading to cardiac failure in those with poor ventricular function
- Acute myocardial infarction post-operatively
- Malignant cardiac arrhythmias, such as fast atrial fibrillation and ventricular tachycardia
- Pulmonary embolism post-operatively
- Positive pressure ventilation: can reduce the venous return
- Metabolic acidosis

What is the most common and 'benign' reason for post-operative oliguria?

The most common cause is due to the physiological 'stress' response to surgery in the first 24–36 h post-operatively. This is due to circulating glucocorticoids and mineralocorticoids inducing salt and water retention. Trauma and various anaesthetic gases also stimulate the release of vasopressin from the posterior pituitary, stimulating a post-operative solute-free water retention.

What signs would you look for when examining a post-operative patient with a low urine output?

- *Dry mouth:* suggests dehydration and an under-filled patient
- *Cool peripheries:* low cardiac output state or sympathetic vasoconstrictive compensation for bleeding or poor fluid resuscitation
- *Pulse:* for arrythmias, and tachycardia suggesting bleeding
- *Blood pressure:* may be too low to provide an adequate renal perfusion pressure. A 'normal' BP of a healthy subject may be too low to provide adequate renal perfusion in a chronically hypertensive patient

- *CVP:* suggestive of under- or over-hydration
- *Palpate for a distended bladder:* the urinary catheter may be blocked
- *Drains:* for bleeding
- *Drug chart* for nephrotoxic agents, e.g. aminoglycosides, non-steroidal anti-inflammatory drugs
- *Fluid balance chart*
- *Urine output chart:* complete anuria output suggests catheter obstruction

What is the main risk of ignoring a poor urine output?

Persisting renal ischaemia, which manifests itself as oliguria may lead to acute tubular necrosis and established acute renal failure. For this reason, post-operative oliguria must be managed in good time.

What investigations would you perform and why?

Investigations serve two main purposes
- To establish the cause for the oliguria
- To determine the effect on the kidney, e.g. is this a reversible problem, or is there established renal failure?

Some investigations:
- *Serum urea and electrolytes:* Elevated creatinine shows decreased renal function, elevated urea is a marker for dehydration
- *Urine sodium and osmolality:* Both are indicators of adequate tubular function
- Other investigations may be performed, e.g. ECG if an MI is suspected, renal ultrasound if obstruction is suspected

How could you tell that the patient has developed acute renal failure?

In the case of oliguria due to acute tubular necrosis, the renal tubules lose their ability to

- Concentrate the urine
- Retain sodium

Thus, certain investigations can be devised to determine if there is tubular dysfunction

	ATN	Pre-renal failure
Urine Na	>20	<40
Urine osmolality	<500	>350
Urine:plasma osmolality ratio	<1.2	>1.2

How would you manage patients with poor urine output?

Management of these patients must be rapid to prevent acute renal failure

- Give the urinary catheter a flush to resolve any obstruction
- Stop nephrotoxic drugs until the state of oliguria has been resolved
- Give a bolus of colloid or crystalloid, e.g. 250–500 ml of gelofusin to determine if adequate filling is required. The response of the CVP to this bolus is also a useful indicator of the circulating volume
- Ensure a good cardiac output, e.g. if the patient is being epicardially paced, the rate may be increased
- If simple measures fail, an inotrope such as dopamine may be introduced, running as an infusion of 3–5 µg/kg/min, or dobutamine

- If the patient is well-filled, small boluses of 10 mg furosemide i.v. may be given, progressing to an infusion
- Inotropes and furosemide, although increasing the urine output, have not shown to reduce the risk of progression to acute renal failure
- Dopamine may not only act to locally increase the renal blood flow, but has a direct inotropic effect, increasing the cardiac output and renal perfusion pressure
- Renal support in the form of dialysis or haemofiltration may also be required

MAGNESIUM BALANCE

M

What is the normal serum level of magnesium?
0.7–1.0 mmol/L.

What is the distribution of magnesium in the body?
Magnesium is the second most abundant intracellular cation after potassium. The total body magnesium is ~25 g, with 65% being located in the bone. Only 1% of the body magnesium is found in the serum, so that the serum level is a poor reflection of the total body store.

What purpose does magnesium serve?
Magnesium is an essential co-factor in a number of enzymes, notably in the transfer of phosphate groups, and protein synthesis. It is most conspicuously important for the normal function of the central nervous, neuromuscular and cardiovascular systems.

What is the relationship between magnesium and serum calcium?
High magnesium levels prevent calcium cellular uptake, and for this reason, hypermagnesaemia can lead to bradycardia and sluggish deep tendon reflexes.

What drug is used to reverse the effects of severe hypermagnesaemia?
Calcium gluconate.

Which organ is largely responsible for magnesium homeostasis?
The kidney is the major site for magnesium balance. It is freely filtered at the glomerulus, and reabsorbed mainly at the proximal convoluted tubule and thick ascending limb of Henle.

What are the main causes of hypomagnesaemia?
- *Renal losses:* any state of excess diuresis, e.g. diuretic use, diuretic phase of acute renal failure, hypercalcemia
- *Alcoholism*

M

- *Gut losses/malabsorption:* diarrhoea, inflammatory bowel disease, malnutrition, intestinal resection and bypasses

- *Endocrine disturbance:* diabetes mellitus, hyperparathyroidism, hyperthyroidism

How common is hypomagnesaemia in the hospital setting?

Hypomagnesaemia occurs in over 60% of the critically ill, most commonly associated with the use of diuretics.

How can hypomagnesaemia be recognised?

It may be difficult to recognise hypomagnesaemia due to its varied presentations. Recognised features include:

- Cardiac arrhythmias such as atrial fibrillation and torsade de pointes (rapid ventricular arrhythmia with a characteristically twisting wave front)

- *ECG changes:* prolonged P-R interval (>220 ms) and widened QRS complex

- Muscular weakness

- Confusion

Give some examples of the therapeutic role of magnesium–containing compounds.

- *Anti-arrhythmic:* can be used to achieve chemical cardioversion for acute atrial fibrillation, or in torsade de pointes

- *Acute myocardial infarction:* some studies suggest a survival benefit from early administration

- *Antacid:* e.g. magnesium trisilicate, or hydroxide

- *Laxative:* e.g. magnesium sulphate

- *Eclampsia:* for the prevention of recurrent seizures in this condition

MECHANICAL VENTILATORY SUPPORT

Give some basic indications for the use of invasive ventilatory support.

The basic effects of mechanical ventilation are improved oxygenation and carbon dioxide elimination. Some of the indications are

- Respiratory rate >35/min, with immanent exhaustion
- Tidal volume <5 ml/kg
- Vital capacity <10–15 ml/kg
- Inadequate oxygenation: PaO_2 < 8 kPa with FiO_2 of >0.6
- Inadequate ventilation with $PaCO_2$ > 8 kPa
- Raised intracranial pressure: keeping the $PaCO_2$ at 4.0–4.5 kPa promotes cerebral vasoconstriction, and hence reduces the intracranial pressure. This may occur at the expense of reducing oxygenation
- Note that the use of ventilation must be appropriate given the prognosis of the disease

Which parameters of ventilation may be adjusted on the mechanical ventilator?

Some parameters that may be adjusted (depending on the type of ventilator used) are

- Respiratory rate
- Tidal volume: 5–7 ml/kg
- Fraction of inspired oxygen (FiO_2): 0.21–1.0
- Flow waveform: a sinusoidal flow during the respiratory cycle reduces the mean airway pressures
- Inspiratory:Expiratory (I:E) ratio: usually 1:2
- Pressure limit
- Addition of PEEP and CPAP: this delivers additional pressure at the end of the cycle

Which parameters need to be adjusted to improve oxygenation?

- Increasing the FiO_2
- Increasing the level of the PEEP
- Increasing the I:E ratio

Which parameters need to be adjusted to improve ventilation?

Ventilation (the ability to 'blow off' CO_2) may be improved by

- Increasing the respiratory rate
- Increasing the tidal volume
- Increasing the peak pressure

What are the basic modes of ventilation?

- *Pressure control:* either a pre-set inspiratory pressure is delivered, or the cycle changes from inspiration to expiration when a certain pressure is reached

- *Volume control:* a fixed tidal volume is delivered, and is generally used by older and simpler circuits

- *Assisted modes:* the ventilator augments each inspiratory effort initiated by the patient – either by pressure or volume support, e.g. PSV (pressure support ventilation), SIMV (synchronised intermittent mandatory ventilation)

What is PEEP (positive end-expiratory pressure), and what physiological changes occur with it?

PEEP is used in conjunction with IPPV, and involves delivery of additional pressure (5–20 cmH$_2$O) at the end of the respirator cycle to prevent alveolar collapse at the end of expiration. Thus, oxygenation is improved when additional alveoli are recruited. Other than alveolar recruitment, some of the other physiological effects are

- Increased compliance
- Increased functional residual capacity (leading to the above)
- Reduced physiological shunting with increased V/Q ratio

Give some examples of the physiological effects and complications of intermittent positive pressure ventilation (IPPV).

- *Cardiovascular:* by making the intrathoracic pressure 'less negative,' it reduces the venous return to the heart. Lung expansion also distorts the alveolar capillaries, increasing the pulmonary vascular resistance. These have the effect of reducing the cardiac output and arterial pressure. Therefore, tissue oxygen delivery may be impaired

- *Respiratory:* overdistension of the lungs produces barotrauma in the form of alveolar rupture. This manifests predominantly as pneumothorax or pneumomediastinum. Also increases the risk of nosocomial pneumonia

- *Renal:* leads to a reduction of the renal perfusion pressure, and hence the urine output

- *Paralytic ileus:* caused by uncertain mechanisms

METABOLIC ACIDOSIS

What is metabolic acidosis?

This is an acid–base disturbance characterised by an increase in the total body acid such that the pH falls below 7.35. There is also a fall of the serum bicarbonate to below the reference range.

In what ways may bicarbonate be lost in cases of metabolic acidosis?

The bicarbonate may be

- Lost from the gut or urine
- Depleted through buffering an overwhelming proton (H^+) load
- Impaired generation of bicarbonate

How may the causes of metabolic acidosis be classified?

The causes may be classified according to the anion gap (*see* 'Acid–base')

$$\text{Anion gap} = (Na^+ + K^+) - (HCO_3^- + Cl^-)$$

Normally, the anion gap is 12–20 mmol/l.

- *Normal anion gap:* the lost bicarbonate is replaced with chloride ions to ensure electro-chemical neutrality. This leads to a characteristic hyperchloraemia. The causes include
    - Gut losses of bicarbonate:
        - Diarrhoea
        - Pancreatic fistula
        - Ileostomy/uretosigmoidostomy
    - Renal losses:
        - Some cases of renal failure
        - Renal tubular acidosis type II
        - Renal tubular acidosis type IV: hypoaldosteronism
- *Increased anion gap:* there is the addition of exogenously or endogenously formed acid that increases the anion gap.

This increased acid load is buffered by circulating bicarbonate, which is then blown off by the lungs as carbon dioxide. Causes include

- Lactic acidosis
- Diabetic ketoacidosis (DKA)
- Some cases of renal failure
- Drugs: salicylates, metformin

What is renal tubular acidosis?

These are a group of conditions that exhibit renal tubular dysfunction in the presence of a normal glomerular filtration rate and creatinine clearance. It leads to abnormalities in the renal handling of H^+ and HCO_3^-. They are classified according to the site of the lesion:

- *Type I (distal):* The most common variety. There is a loss in the ability to excrete acid at the collecting ducts, leading to acidosis
- *Type II (proximal):* There is a reduction of proximal tubular bicarbonate absorptive capacity, leading to loss of bicarbonate. It may be seen in Fanconi's syndrome
- *Type IV:* There is a hyperkalaemic acidosis resulting from hypoaldosteronism

What effects can acidosis have on body physiology?

- Shift of the oxygen dissociation curve to the right, signifying a reduction of the haemoglobin molecule's oxygen affinity. Therefore, there is an increased tendency to oxygenate the tissues
- Decreased myocardial contractility
- Resistance to the effects of circulating catecholamines
- *Pulmonary hypertension:* acidosis causes pulmonary vasoconstriction
- *Cardiac arrhythmias:* both as a direct effect, and through the development of hyperkalaemia
- Increased sympathetic activity, with a paradoxical catecholamine resistance

What term is given to the tachypnoea of metabolic acidosis?

Kussmaul's respiration.

What are the principles of management of any cause of metabolic acidosis?

The principles of management involve

- Assessment of the severity of the acidosis and the attendant complications on the organ systems mentioned above
- Management of the underlying causes, e.g. fluids/insulin for DKA, emergency dialysis for renal failure
- *Bicarbonate therapy:* this is a controversial issue. If it is to be used in severe cases, it is more justified in cases of hyperchloraemic metabolic acidosis where the primary problem is a loss of bicarbonate (*see* 'Lactic acidosis')

METABOLIC ALKALOSIS

What is the essential disturbance that defines a metabolic alkalosis?

The essential change is a primary increase in the serum bicarbonate to above 30 mmol/l.

Which ions other than bicarbonate are implicated in the development of metabolic alkalosis?

The other ions are

- *Hydrogen ions (protons):* loss of protons (e.g. by vomiting) leads to a compensatory increase in bicarbonate and hence alkalosis

- *Chloride:* loss of this ion causes the renal tubules to increase bicarbonate uptake in order to maintain electrochemical neutrality. Note that there is a close relationship between bicarbonate and chloride: the loss of one leads to gain of the other

- *Potassium:* loss of potassium leads to increased absorption of bicarbonate in the renal tubules. Also leads to increased cellular uptake of protons

Which organ system is most commonly involved in metabolic alkalosis?

Gut pathology is often implicated.

Give some examples of the causes of metabolic alkalosis.

- *Addition of bicarbonate to the system:*
  - Iatrogenic administration
  - Milk–alkali syndrome
- *Loss of chloride (with gain of bicarbonate):*
  - Persistent vomiting
  - Mucus-secreting adenoma (also loss of potassium)
  - Diuretics

- *Any cause of hypokalaemia:* causing a shift of protons into the cell
- *'Contraction' alkalosis:* volume depletion is associated with increased bicarbonate absorption over chloride

Describe the mechanism by which metabolic alkalosis develops in cases of pyloric stenosis.

In the case of pyloric stenosis – either acquired or congenital, metabolic alkalosis develops and is perpetuated by normal compensatory mechanisms

- Gastric acid is a rich source of protons and chloride, which are both lost in the vomitus
- There is a reduction of pancreatic juice secretion due to reduced acid load at the duodenum. Pancreatic juice contains a lot of bicarbonate, which is therefore retained
- Volume depletion maintains the alkalosis by leading to bicarbonate absorption over chloride
- There is increased uptake of bicarbonate at renal tubules in (response to a loss of chloride) in order to maintain electrochemical neutrality

Why may patients with metabolic alkalosis develop poor tissue oxygenation?

There are two main reasons

- As part of the body's compensatory response to alkalosis, there is hypoventilation in order to increase the $PaCO_2$
- Alkalosis causes a shift of the oxygen dissociation curve to the *left* signifying increased haemoglobin affinity for oxygen, at the expense of tissue oxygen uptake

NUTRITION: BASIC CONCEPTS

Describe how the state of nutrition may be assessed.

There are many methods of assessing the nutritional state – none of them completely satisfactory.

- Anthropometric measures
  - Height, weight, body mass index (Weight/Height^2)
  - Fat measure indices: e.g. triceps skin fold thickness
  - Lean muscle indices: e.g. mid-arm circumference
- Biochemical indices
  - *Serum proteins:* e.g. albumin; more of a late marker because of the long half life. Other states of critical illness may also affect the level. Other proteins that have been measured: pre-albumin, transferrin, retinol, all of which may be affected by the stress response
  - *24 h urinary creatinine:* as a measure of the protein turnover
- Immunological indices
  - Total lymphocyte count
  - Immune function, e.g. tuberculin skin test, response to mitogens. However, these are non-specific
- Clinical markers
  - Physical appearance
  - Hand grip strength
  - Pulmonary function tests, e.g. vital capacity

From which sources may the energy requirements be satisfied? How much energy do each of these provide?

The predominant sources of energy are from carbohydrates and lipid, but protein catabolism also yields energy.

- Fats provide 9.3 kcal/g of energy
- Glucose, 4.1 kcal/g
- Protein, 4.1 kcal/g

Define the respiratory quotient.

This is defined as 'the ratio of the volume of the CO_2 produced to the volume of oxygen consumed for the oxidation of a given amount of nutrient.'

Respiratory quotients for the oxidation of nutrients
- Carbohydrate: 1.0
- Fat: 0.70
- Protein: 0.80

What are the disadvantages of using glucose as the main energy source? How can this be overcome?

The problems of glucose are
- As part of the stress response, the critically ill are often in a state of hyperglycaemia and glucose intolerant. Therefore, if glucose is the only source of energy, then patients will not receive their required daily amount due to poor utilisation of their energy source
- The excess glucose occurring as a consequence of the above is converted to lipid in the liver, leading to fatty change. This may derange the liver function tests
- The extra CO_2 released upon oxidation of the glucose may lead to respiratory failure and increased ventilatory requirements
- Relying solely on glucose may lead to a deficiency of the essential fatty acids

Therefore, at least 50% of the total energy requirement must be provided by fat. Too little glucose leads to hypoglycaemia and stimulation of ketogenesis.

What is the recommended daily intake of protein and nitrogen?

The recommended daily intake of protein is 0.8 g/kg/day, and that of nitrogen is 0.15 g/kg/day. Note that these values increase in the catabolic state of critical illness.

How much protein provides 1 g of nitrogen?

6.25 g of protein yields 1 g of nitrogen.

What is an 'essential' amino acid? Give examples

The essential amino acids are those ones that cannot be synthesised in the body and have to be ingested in the diet. These include: leucine, isoleucine, lysine, methionine, phenylalanine, threonine, tryptophan and valine.

Give some examples of essential minerals.

Zinc, magnesium, manganese, selenium, copper, chromium and molybdenum.

What are the fat-soluble vitamins, and what are they used for?

- *Vitamin A:* important for cell membrane stabilisation and retinal function

- *Vitamin D:* for calcium homeostasis and bone mineralisation

- *Vitamin E (mainly α tocopherol):* acts as a free radical scavenger

- *Vitamin K:* involved in the γ carboxylation of glutamic acid residues of factors II, VII, IX and X during blood coagulation

What are the names of the vitamin B group?
Which diseases occur when there is a deficiency?

The B group of vitamins, which are all water-soluble are composed of

- *Vitamin B₁ (thiamine):* deficiency leads to beri-beri or Weinicke's encephalopathy

- *Vitamin B₂ (riboflavin):* deficiency leads to a syndrome of glossitis, angular stomatitis and cheilosis

- *Vitamin B₃ (niacin):* deficiency leads to pellegra

- *Biotin:* deficiency rarely occurs in isolation, but can lead to reduced immune function

- *Vitamin B_6 (pyridoxine):* deficiency leads to stomatitis and peripheral neuropathy
- *Vitamin B_{12} (cobalamin) and folate:* deficiency produces megaloblastic anaemia

What are the functions of vitamin C?

Vitamin C is another of the water-soluble vitamins

- Hydroxylation of proline and lysine residues during collagen synthesis
- Iron absorption at the gut
- Synthesis of epinephrine from tyrosine
- Antioxidant functions

OXYGEN: BASIC PHYSIOLOGY

How is oxygen transported in the body?

Oxygen is transported by binding to haemoglobin (99%), or dissolved in solution (1%).

What does Henry's law state, and how is this used to calculate the amount of oxygen dissolved in the blood?

Henry's law states that the gas content of a solution is equal to the product of the solubility and the partial pressure of the gas. In the case of oxygen, at 37°C, the solubility is 0.03 ml/L for every mmHg rise in the partial pressure.

Therefore the amount of oxygen dissolved in the blood is $0.03 \times PaO_2$.

What is haemoglobin composed of?

Haemoglobin is a globular protein consisting of a haem component and a globin chain.

The haem moeity consists of Fe^{2+} and a protoporphyrin ring.

In the adult, the globin chain consists of 2-α and 2-β chains together with a 2,3 bisphosphoglycerate (2,3 BPG) molecule.

A total of 4 oxygen molecules (i.e. 8 atoms) are able to bind to each haemoglobin molecule.

Apart from oxygen, what other molecules may bind to haemoglobin under normal circumstances?

- *Carbon dioxide:* This binds to the globin chain, forming a carbamino compound
- *Protons (H^+):* These bind to the globin chain, specifically to amino, carboxyl and imidazole groups
- *2,3 BPG:* This is a by-product of red cell metabolism. It is able to form covalent bonds with the beta subunits, wedging them apart in the de-oxygenated state

Where are the main sites of haemopoesis?

- *Bone marrow:* from the first few weeks after birth
- *Liver and spleen:* most important sites up until the first 7 months of gestation. The adult can revert to these sites in pathological states – so-called 'extramedullary haemopoesis'
- *Yolk sac:* in the first few weeks of gestation

What is the life span of the red cell?

120 days, after which it is broken down by the reticulo-endothelial system.

Draw the oxygen dissociation curve, and label the axes.

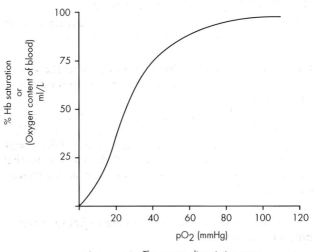

The oxygen dissociation curve

What accounts for the shape of the curve?

The sigmoidal curve reflects the progressive nature with which each oxygen molecule binds to haemoglobin. This binding is termed cooperative – the binding of one oxygen facilitates the binding of the next.

What is the Bohr effect, and what causes it?

The Bohr effect is a shift of the dissociation curve to the *right,* signifying a reduction of the oxygen affinity of the molecule, and therefore a greater tendency to off-load oxygen into the tissues. It is brought about by

- Increased temperature
- Increased acidity
- Increased 2,3 BPG (e.g. due to chronic hypoxia)
- Hypercarbia

What physiological effect does it have?

It ensures greater and more ready tissue oxygenation in states an acute or chronic reduction of tissue perfusion.

How does the oxygen dissociation curve in the fetus compare to that of the adult, and what accounts for this difference?

The fetal oxygen-dissociation curve is shifted to the *left,* reflecting the increased oxygen affinity of fetal haemoglobin caused by the presence of the γ subunit (instead of the β) that cannot form covalent bonds with 2,3 BPG. This ensures that it is able to readily take up oxygen from the maternal haemoglobin molecule.

How much oxygen is bound to haemoglobin when fully saturated?

When fully saturated, each gram of haemoglobin can bind to 1.34 ml of oxygen. It follows that, the oxygen-carrying capacity of the blood is 1.34 × [Hb] at full (100%) saturation.

Bearing this in mind, on what factors does the total amount of oxygen in the blood depend? How is this calculated?

$$\frac{\text{Total O}_2 \text{ content}}{\text{of blood}} = \frac{\text{Amount bound to Hb}}{+ \text{ amount dissolved in blood}}$$

or,

$$= (1.34 \times [\text{Hb}] \times \% \text{ saturation}) + (0.03 \times \text{PaO}_2)$$

Therefore, the factors determining the total oxygen content of the blood are

- Haemoglobin concentration
- Percent saturation of the molecule
- Partial pressure of oxygen
- Temperature: This determines the oxygen solubility (although this is in practice of little significance)

The total is in the order of 200 ml/L for arterial blood at 97% saturation.

OXYGEN THERAPY

How may oxygen be delivered to the patient?

- *Variable performance devices:* the FiO_2 delivered depends on the flow rate.
  - *Nasal cannulae:* a convenient way for the patient
  - *Face mask (e.g. Hudson mask):* at 2 l/min, the FiO_2 achieved is 0.25–0.30. At 6–10 l/min: $FiO_2 = 0.30–0.40$

    If the flow is not high enough, then re-breathing of air exhaled into the mask occurs, leading to hypercarbia.

- *Fixed performance devices:* there is a constant FiO_2 delivered so the desired amount can be administered accurately.
  - *Venturi mask:* oxygen flows through a device that entrains air from side holes at a certain rate. The degree of air mixing within the device produces the desired FiO_2
  - *Reservoir bag:* this is attached onto the end of a face mask. During tachypnoea, the patient inhales directly from the oxygen in the bag, so that the FiO_2 is close to 1.0. This is used in the trauma setting to deliver as much oxygen as possible
  - *Oxygen tent*
  - *Continuous positive pressure ventilation:* this ensures that the small airways do not collapse at the end of expiration by providing a positive pressure through the respiratory cycle
  - *Invasive respiratory support* with intubation and intermittent positive pressure ventilation

What is the danger of oxygen therapy in the chronic CO_2-retaining patient and what is the pathophysiology?

In the patient who is chronically retaining CO_2, uncontrolled use of oxygen may induce apnoea. There are two main explanations

- Loss of hypoxic pulmonary drive. Those who have a chronically raised CO_2 rely on hypoxia to stimulate respiration. If this is abolished by the use of oxygen, then apnoea may be the result. To prevent this, the patient must initially be given 24% oxygen which is steadily increased depending on the effect

- Abolition of hypoxia can reverse the normal compensatory hypoxic pulmonary vasoconstriction. This leads to worsening V/Q mismatch

What are the other potential problems associated with oxygen therapy?

- *Absorption atelectasis:* in the absence of nitrogen (which by its slow absorption 'splints' the airway open), oxygen is absorbed rapidly from the alveolus, causing the airway to collapse after it

- *Pulmonary toxicity:* oxygen irritates the mucosa of the airways directly, leading to loss of surfactant and progressive fibrosis

- *Retinopathy* by retrolenticular fibroplasia

- *Risk of fires and explosions:* oxygen supports combustion

PARENTERAL NUTRITION (TPN)

P

What are the indications for TPN?

- General critical illness:
  - Severe malnourishment with >10% loss of weight
  - Multiple trauma
  - Sepsis/multisystem failure
  - Severe burns
- Gut problems:
  - Enterocutaneous fistula
  - Short bowel syndrome
  - Inflammatory bowel disease
  - Radiation enteritis

Which is the absolute indication for TPN?

The most important indication is the presence of an enterocutaneous fistula.

How is TPN administered?

The high osmolality of the mixture causes irritation to small vessels, so that it is generally given through a central vein, e.g. tunnelled subclavian line. If it is to be given through a peripheral vein, it must be given as a solution of osmolality of <900 mOsm/l.

What are the basic components of a TPN regimen?

The basic components are water, carbohydrate, protein, lipid, vitamin and trace elements. Various drugs may also be added, such as ranitidine and insulin.

How is TPN monitored?

Monitoring involves nutritional status and biochemical markers
- More than once per day:
  - Glucose

▼ 171

- Once per day:
  - Serum electrolytes
  - Urea and creatinine
- Twice-weekly check:
  - Albumin and total protein
  - Calcium
  - Magnesium
  - Phosphate
  - Liver function tests

Why does liver function need to be monitored?

TPN can cause a derangement of the liver function tests secondary to enzyme induction caused by amino acid imbalances. Also, it can cause fatty change of the liver.

What are the metabolic complications?

- Hyper/hypoglycaemia
- Hyperlipidaemia
- Essential fatty acid deficiency
- Hyperchloraemic metabolic acidosis: if there is an excess of chloride
- Hyperammoniaemia: if there is liver disease, or a deficiency of L-glutamine and arginine
- Ventilatory problems: with excess production of CO_2 if too much glucose is used in the mixture. In the ventilated critically ill patient, the amount of glucose given in 24 h may have to be restricted to 5 g/kg

PNEUMONIA

What are the normal respiratory defence mechanisms?

- Nasal humidification of inhaled air
- Airway mucus secretion
- Intact cough reflex
- Mucociliary action of respiratory epithelium
- Alveolar macrophages
- Secretory IgA

What is the definition of pneumonia?

Pneumonia is an inflammatory condition of the lung char-acterised by consolidation due to the presence of exudate in the alveolar spaces.

What are the pathological types of pneumonia?

- *Lobar pneumonia:* the exudate forms directly in the bronchioles and alveoli and spills over into adjacent segments via the pores of Kohn. The consolidation is sharply confined to a particular lobe. It is typically pneumococcal in origin

- *Bronchopneumonia:* the inflammatory process starts at the bronchioles and extends to the alveoli, leading to numerous foci of consolidation. It is more common at the extremes of age, and in those with chronic illness

- *Interstitial pneumonia:* consists of a group of conditions characterised by chronic alveolar inflammation, which are not necessarily infective in origin and may have an immunological basis

What are the classical pathological phases of lobar pneumonia?

There are four pathologically recognised stages

- *Acute congestion (day 1–2):* the lobe is heavy, dark and firm with inflammatory exudate and cellular infiltrate, including erythrocytes

- *Red hepatisation (day 2–4):* the lung is firm, red and consolidated. The alveolar spaces contain neutrophils, fibrin and extravasated erythrocytes

- *Grey hepatisation (day 4–8):* the lobe is heavy, consolidated and grey. There is an extensive fibrin network with degenerating erythrocytes

- *Resolution (>day 8):* macrophage action liquefies the exudate with fibrinolytic enzymes. Full resolution may take up to 3 weeks

How common is pneumonia in the ITU and which organisms are involved?

Nosocomial pneumonia in the ITU may occur in 30–40% of ventilated patients and 15–20% of the unventilated.

Ventilator-associated pneumonia may be divided into early onset (1–4 days following intubation) and late onset (beyond day 4).

Organisms involved

- *Early onset:* Oropharyngeal organisms mainly e.g. *Strep. pneumoniae, Staph. aureus* (including MRSA), *Haemophilus influenzae*

- *Late onset:* Usually involving Gram negative organisms, e.g. *Pseudomonas* spp., *Enterobacter, Acinetobacter*

What are the risk factors for nosocomial pneumonia in the intubated patient?

- Loss of anatomic barriers due to instrumentation: organisms can enter the lower respiratory tract when the epiglottis and glottis are breached by the endotracheal tube

- Impaired cough reflex: as the endotracheal tube opens the glottis

- Re-intubation
- Colonisation of other instruments, e.g. tubing in the ventilator circuit, and Y-connectors for tubing
- Aspiration of gastric contents which may be colonised by bacteria
- Prone positioning predisposes to aspiration
- Epithelial trauma to the airway, e.g. by suction devices
- Cross colonisation from staff and other patients
- Generalised debilitating or chronic illness, e.g. malignancy, diabetes mellitus, burns, general trauma, and uraemia

Which factors predispose the stomach to bacterial colonisation?

The risk of bacterial colonisation increases when the gastric pH > 4.0

- Use of H_2-blockers to prevent stress ulceration
- Continuous gastric feeding
- Chronic atrophic gastritis leading to achlorhydria

How is pneumonia recognised in the ITU setting?

The 'Gold Standard' for the diagnosis of pneumonia in the ITU is direct biopsy of suspected lung tissue, but this is not ideal.

Many of the clinical features are common to a number of conditions, such as atelectasis.

Features include

- New or progressing pulmonary infiltrates
- Pyrexia >38°C
- Leucocytosis >14,000
- Purulent tracheal secretions
- Positive Gram staining and cultures in the light of these changes
- Specimens may be collected by:
  - Bronchio-alveolar lavage
  - Brushing

- Trans-thoracic needle biopsy
- Open/video-assisted lung biopsy

How can pneumonia be prevented?

Prevention is always more effective than prolonged antibiotic treatment. This involves

- Protective isolation of high-risk patients
- Control of cross infection by staff, e.g. hand-washing
- Intermittent, and not continuous enteral feeding
- Controlled use of antibiotics to prevent multi-drug resistance
- Use of sucralfate for stress ulcer prophylaxis
- Suctioning of sub-glottic secretions
- Decreasing the number of times that the ventilator circuit is 'broken' by connections

What are the complications of bacterial pneumonia?

Complications include

- Pleuritis: leading to pleural effusion and healing with extensive adhesions
- Empyema: a loculated collection of pus in the pleural cavity surrounded by a fibrinous wall
- Lung abscess formation, which can erode to form a broncho-pleural fistula
- Metastatic abscesses, e.g. cerebral abscess
- Generalised sepsis

PNEUMOTHORAX

What types of pneumothorax are there, and what are their identifying features?

There are three types of pneumothorax

- *Simple pneumothorax:* where there is air in the pleural space, but no cardiovascular compromise

- *Tension pneumothorax:* there is a one–way valve effect that allows air to enter the pleural space, but not to leave it. Mediastinal shift and compression from the air in the pleural space displaces the heart and great vessels, producing cardiovascular compromise and shock

- *Open pneumothorax ('sucking chest wound'):* an open defect in the thoracic wall draws in air during the respiratory cycle, leading to tension pneumothorax

Note that a simple pneumothorax, if left unmanaged may lead to tension pneumothorax when large enough to cause mediastinal shift.

What are the causes of pneumothorax?

Some causes are

- *Spontaneous pneumothorax:* following the rupture of apical blebs of unknown origin. Also occurs more commonly in asthma, cystic fibrosis, or associated with bullous disease in COPD

- *Traumatic:* with both blunt and penetrating chest injury

- *Iatrogenic:* e.g. following pleural aspiration, central line insertion, oesophagoscopy and barotrauma from IPPV

What are the signs on clinical examination?

For simple pneumothorax:

- Ipsilateral reduction of chest wall movements
- Increased resonance to percussion
- Reduced breath sounds
- Occasionally, the presence of subcutaneous emphysema
- Tachycardia: a non-specific sign

With tension pneumothorax, there is the above, together with

- Tracheal deviation indicating mediastinal shift to the opposite side
- Hypotension
- Elevated CVP
- Cyanosis despite tachypnoea

How may pneumothorax be recognised in the mechanically ventilated patient?

- Sudden increase in the inflation pressure
- Sudden and unexplained hypoxia
- Development of a new cardiac arrhythmia, such as atrial fibrillation
- Sudden hypotension or rising CVP

How is the diagnosis of pneumothorax confirmed?

A chest radiograph taken during expiration confirms the diagnosis. Tension pneumothorax is a clinical diagnosis that must be managed by life-saving chest decompression before waiting for the radiograph to confirm.

How is pneumothorax managed?

- All types require the airway to be secured, together with administration of 100% oxygen by face mask
- Tension pneumothorax is managed by emergency needle decompression
- Ultimately, chest tube thoracostomy is required once the tension has been converted to a simple pneumothorax following decompression. This also drains blood in traumatic cases
- For an open pneumothorax, an occlusive dressing is applied to the surface of the wound, being taped down on three sides. This acts as a one-way valve, allowing air to escape on expiration, and preventing air entry on inspiration

- Recurrent cases of spontaneous pneumothorax may be managed by open or thoracoscopic pleurectomy. By stripping the parietal pleura, adhesions form between the lung and chest wall, preventing further collapse

How is emergency decompression of a tension pneumothorax carried out?

- The patient is administered 100% oxygen
- A large bore (14 or 16-guage) needle is inserted into the 2nd intercosal space in the mid–clavicular line. It must pass along the upper border of the third rib to prevent injury to the neuro–vascular bundle
- The correct position is confirmed by the presence of the hissing sound of escaping air
- A chest tube thoracostomy is prepared for definitive management

POTASSIUM BALANCE

What is the normal level of the serum potassium?
3.5–5.0 mmol/l.

What is the distribution of potassium in the body?
98% of the total body potassium is intracellular. The intracellular concentration is ~150 mmol/l compared to ~4 mmol/l in the serum.

How is potassium regulated?
There are a number of influential factors on serum potassium

- *Dietary potassium:* the 'Western' diet may contain 20–100 mmol of potassium daily

- *Aldosterone:* this is a mineralocorticoid steroid hormone produced by the zona glomerulosa of the adrenal cortex. It stimulates sodium reabsorption in the distal convoluted tubule and cortical collecting duct through an active exchange with potassium, whose excretion is therefore promoted

- *Acid-Base balance:* potassium and H^+ are exchanged at the cell membrane, so that excess of one or the other leads to increased exchange. Thus, acidosis leads to hyperkalaemia and vice versa. Similarly, alkalosis can lead to hypokalaemia and vice versa. This also occurs at the kidney where reabsorption of one causes excretion of the other

- *Tubular fluid flow rate:* increased flow rate promotes potassium secretion. This is one method by which some diuretics may cause hypokalaemia

- *Insulin:* this stimulates potassium uptake into cells, reducing the serum level

What are the causes of hyperkalaemia?
- Artefact: haemolysis in the blood bottle
- Excess oral or i.v. administration

- Redistribution:
  - Between the ICF and ECF due to injury: intravascular haemolysis, burns, tissue necrosis
  - Reduced cellular uptake: insulin deficiency, acidosis
- Decreased excretion:
  - Renal origin: renal failure, potassium-sparing diuretics
  - Adrenal origin: Addison's disease
  - Mineralocorticoid resistance: systemic lupus erythematosus, chronic interstitial nephritis

What ECG changes may be found in hyper- and hypokalaemia?

- In hyperkalaemia:
  - Tall, tented T-waves
  - Small P-waves
  - Wide QRS-complexes
- In hypokalaemia:
  - Small/inverted T-waves
  - U-waves (seen after the T-waves)
  - Prolonged P-R interval
  - S-T segment depression

What is the emergency management of hyperkalaemia?

Before any treatment is instituted, the serum potassium must be rechecked to determine if it is a spurious finding. If it comes back as >6.5 mmol/l, then

- Commence continuous cardiac monitoring
- Calcium gluconate or calcium chloride (10%) is given by slow i.v. route for membrane-stabilisation
- Insulin with 5% dextrose infusion is commenced to increase intracellular uptake of potassium
- Ion exchange resin therapy with oral or rectal calcium resonium can be used

- Bicarbonate (50–100 mmol/l) may be given to correct acidosis, and further increase cellular uptake of potassium
- Haemodialysis if the potassium is persistently high, or there is severe acidosis (pH < 7.20)

What use does knowledge of the cardiac effects of potassium have for surgical practice?

It is well known that hyperkalaemia can cause the heart to arrest in diastole. Knowledge of this has permitted the development of potassium-rich cardioplegic solutions used to arrest the heart in diastole to permit cardiac surgery.

What are the causes of hypokalaemia?

- Artefact: Drip arm sampling
- Redistribution
  - Between the ECF and ICF: alkalosis, insulin excess
- Decreased oral intake: Starvation (this is rare)
- Loss from body:
  - GIT losses: vomiting, diarrhoea, entero–cutaneous fistulae, mucin-secreting adenomas of the colon
  - Renal losses: Conn's and Cushing's syndromes, diuretics (e.g. loop and thiazides), renal tubular acidosis

What are the clinical features associated with hypokalaemia?

- Muscular weakness and cramps
- Lethargy and confusion
- Atrial and ventricular arrhythmias
- Increased digoxin toxicity
- Paralytic ileus

PULMONARY ARTERY CATHETER

Define the cardiac output.

The cardiac output is the product of the heart rate and the stroke volume. It is in the order of 5–6 l/min.

Define the cardiac index.

The cardiac index is the cardiac output divided by the body surface area. The minimum acceptable level for adequate tissue perfusion is 2.2–2.5 l/min/m².

What is a pulmonary artery catheter and what purpose does it serve?

This is a multi-lumen, balloon-tipped, flow-directed catheter that is passed through the right heart and into the pulmonary artery.

In certain instances, it provides a more useful picture of left heart function than CVP measures alone, and can be used to calculate a number of useful parameters of cardiovascular function in the critically ill, thus providing both severity assessment and therapeutic guidance.

By which principle does it reflect left heart function?

When 'wedged' in a branch of the pulmonary artery (balloon inflated in a branch of the PA), there is a continuous column of blood beyond the tip of the catheter that extends to the left atrium. Thus, the pulmonary artery pressure at the 'wedged' position is equal to the left atrial pressure.

Give some indications for its use.

The indications for its use are controversial, variable and not absolute

- Concomitant with the use of inotropic support, especially vasodilators
- Post-cardiac surgery in those with poor left ventricular function and pulmonary hypertension
- Those with suspected ARDS and pulmonary oedema

- Shock of any cause, e.g. assessing the systemic vascular resistance in those with septic shock
- Those with multi-organ failure
- Multiple injury with thoracic injury

What physiological parameters does it measure directly?
- Mean arterial pressure (MAP)
- Heart rate
- Mean pulmonary artery pressure (MPAP)
- Cardiac output (CO)
- Pulmonary artery occlusion pressure (PAOP)
- Ejection fraction
- Mixed venous oxygen saturation

What are the derived variables?
- Cardiac index (cardiac output/body surface area)
- Stroke volume
- Systemic vascular resistance (SVR)
- Pulmonary vascular resistance (PVR)
- Indexed SVR and PVR (these values divided by the Body Surface Area)
- Oxygen delivery and oxygen consumption

Define the systemic vascular resistance.

$$\text{The systemic vascular resistance} = \frac{\text{MAP} - \text{CVP}}{\text{CO}} \times 80.$$

The normal range is $900-1400 \, \text{dyn/s/cm}^{-5}$.

Define the pulmonary vascular resistance.

$$\text{The pulmonary vascular resistance} = \frac{\text{MPAP} - \text{PAOP}}{\text{CO}} \times 80.$$

The normal range is $150-250 \, \text{dyn/s/cm}^{-5}$.

Draw and label a graph of the pressure waveforms encountered as the catheter if floated into position.

Tracing of pressures during passage of the pulmonary artery catheter from the internal jugular vein into the pulmonary artery

A, atrial contraction; V, ventricular contraction
Adapted from Mathay M A. Clin Chest Med 1983; **4**: 233

Diagram taken from Article
"Monitoring & inotropes in the ICU" by
Charles Schmulian in the journal "Surgery Vol. 16: 4 p 78–84 (April 1998)
Published by the "Medicine Publishing Co Ltd" ISSN 0263 9319

What are the complications of insertion?

- Those complications of any central line insertion: *see* 'Central line insertion'
- Cardiac arrhythmias: most commonly atrial and ventricular ectopics. Ventricular tachycardia and ventricular fibrillation as well as heart block also reported
- Cardiac valve injury: leading to incompetence of the tricuspid or pulmonary valves
- Pulmonary artery rupture: this presents as shock and haemoptysis. Occurs from injury by the J-wire, or following balloon inflation
- Pulmonary infarction: if the balloon is kept in the wedged position for too long. Also occurs if there is embolisation

of a thrombus formed at the catheter tip, or catheter migration

- Catheter knotting
- Sepsis

By which principle is the cardiac output measured?

The cardiac output is measured using the indicator dilution or the thermodilution techniques. Both of these have similar principles. With the indicator dilution technique, indocyanine green is injected into the circulation and samples are taken peripherally from the radial artery. A graph of the concentration of the dye in the peripheral blood over time is plotted. The cardiac output equates to the amount of dye injected divided by the area under the curve.

In the case of the thermodilution method, 10 ml of cold crystalloid is injected peripherally, and the change of temperature detected by a thermistor at the end of the catheter. A graph is also plotted for the change of temperature of the blood passing the thermistor against time. This graph is used to calculate the cardiac output.

PULMONARY THROMBOEMBOLISM

What are the risk factors for deep venous thrombosis (DVT)?

- Increased age
- Venous stasis from immobilisation:
  - Prolonged bed rest
  - Recent surgery
  - Cardiac failure
  - Polycythemia: causing increased blood viscosity
- General medical illness:
  - Malignancy
  - Dehydration, including the nephrotic syndrome
  - General sepsis
- Vessel injury: multiple/lower limb injury
- Haematological propensity:
  - Protein C/protein S deficiency
  - Antithrombin III deficiency
  - Factor V Leyden
  - Antiphospholipid antibodies
  - HRT and the oral contraceptive pill

Note that in any one individual, the risk factors are often multiple.

Where do the thrombi commonly form?

They commonly form within the deep veins of the calf, or the deep plexus of veins at the soleus muscle. They may also occur more proximally at the external and common iliac veins, extending to the inferior vena cava. Beyond this, they may also form in the right atrium, acting as a source of pulmonary embolism in atrial fibrillation.

How may a DVT present?

- Painless or painful leg swelling: tenderness at the calf may also be present
- Phlegmasia cerulea dolens: an acutely ischaemic and cyanotic leg following a massive ileo-femoral venous thrombosis
- Phlegmasia alba dolens: an acutely ischaemic, swollen white leg following massive ileo-femoral DVT with arterial spasm
- Pulmonary embolism

How can pulmonary thromboembolism be prevented?

- Peri-operative use of heparin: may be given subcutaneously or as an infusion
- Thromboembolic (TED) stockings
- Intermittent pneumatic compression: which can be used intra-operatively
- Early ambulation of patients
- Transvenous intracaval device: such as umbrella and wire filters, which can be inserted under local anaesthesia to prevent recurrent emboli

How may a pulmonary embolus (PE) present?

Pulmonary emboli may present in a number of ways, depending on the size, number and chronicity of the event

- Sudden cardiac death or cardiac arrest with pulseless electrical activity
- Tachycardia and tachypnoea, with or without pleuritic chest pain
- In the case of massive PE, the patient develops shock due to obstruction to right ventricular outflow. There is a low cardiac index manifest as cool, pale peripheries and systemic hypotension

- There may be evidence of an elevated right ventricular afterload – with a widely split second heart sound with a loud pulmonary component. There may also be a third or fourth heart sounds and functional tricuspid regurgitation
- In the presence of pulmonary infarction, there is a pleural rub
- Chronic, multiple emboli can present with secondary pulmonary hypertension and cor pulmonale
- Paradoxical embolisation can occur through a patent foramen ovale, presenting with systemic embolisation

What is the pathophysiology of a PE?

There is pulmonary artery obstruction as the embolus impacts in a vascular branch beyond the right ventricular outflow tract. There is also the release of vasoacive mediators from activated platelets within the thrombus. Both of these factors conspire to increase the pulmonary vascular resistance and right ventricular afterload. This produces ventricular strain, manifesting as tachycardia.

Reduced flow to lung units causes a V/Q mismatch and increased physiological dead space. This may occur with a bronchospasm induced by circulating mediators. Consequently, there is hypoxia, hypocarbia with tachypnoea.

List the investigations that can be used to make a diagnosis of a PE.

- ECG
- Chest radiograph: more helpful in excluding differential diagnoses
- Arterial blood gas analysis: the V/Q mismatch is seen as hypoxia and hypocarbia
- Plasma D–dimer levels: elevated
- Ventilation–perfusion scan
- Spiral CT scan
- Pulmonary angiography: the 'Gold Standard'

What are the most common ECG changes, and why do these changes occur?

The most common ECG change, apart from sinus tachycardia, is T-wave inversion in the anterior leads.

This may represent reciprocal changes arising from inferior/posterior ischaemia occurring when a pressure-overloaded right ventricle compresses the right coronary artery.

What is a D-dimer, and how useful a diagnostic investigation is this?

D-dimer is a fibrin–degradation product formed by the action of plasmin on the fibrin clot. It may be measured by a latex agglutination test or enzyme linked immunosorbent assay (ELISA). It misses 10% of those with a PE.

How are PEs managed?

This involves initial resuscitation, followed by medical or surgical intervention

- During cardiopulmonary resuscitation, a precordial thump may help to dislodge an obstructing mass
- Thrombolysis: with thrombolytic agents may be used in those who are haemodynamically unstable following a large embolus, e.g. streptokinase and urokinase can be infused directly into the pulmonary artery
- Following this, anticoagulation with heparin and warfarin is required
- Pulmonary embolectomy: this can be performed either as an open technique, or using a catheter. These methods are also reserved for the haemodynamically unstable

What is the mechanism of action of heparin?

Heparin augments the activity of antithrombin III, an inhibitor of activated factors IX, X, XI and XII, preventing the conversion of fibrinogen to fibrin.

▼

What is the mechanism of action of warfarin?

Warfarin prevents the reduction of vitamin K epoxide to vitamin K, thereby inhibiting the vitamin K-dependant binding of factors II, VII, IX and X to calcium and phospholipid membrane surfaces during the clotting cascade.

P

PULSE OXIMETRY

What is pulse oximetry, and what does it measure?

Pulse oximetry is a non-invasive and continuous method of assessing arterial oxygen saturation (SaO_2) and pulse rate.

Note that it is not a measure of the total oxygen content of the blood nor the PaO_2. It does not assess ventilation, which requires a measure of the $PaCO_2$.

By which principle does pulse oximetry work?

Pulse oximetry works on the principles of spectrophotometry. It contains a probe emitting light at the red (660 nm) and infra-red (940 nm) wavelengths, and a photodetector.

It relies on the differing amount of light absorbed by the saturated and unsaturated Hb molecules. The percentage oxygen saturation of the blood is calculated from the ratio of these two forms of the molecule.

What are its disadvantages and sources of error?

Problems encountered include

- Diminished accuracy below a saturation of ~70%
- There is a delay of ~20 s between actual and displayed values, limiting its use in the emergency setting
- Poor peripheral perfusion leads to a poor signal quality
- So does ambient light pollution
- Abnormal pigments affect the results. External pigments include nail varnish. Internal pigments include bilirubin of the jaundiced patient, methaemoglobin, and carboxyhaemoglobin. Jaundice underestimates the true SaO_2 and carbon monoxide poisoning overestimates the true SaO_2
- Abnormal pulsations, such as cardiac arrhythmia or venous pulsations of right heart valve defects may interfere with the signal
- Note, however, that there is no interference from polycythemia or fetal haemoglobin

▼

What is methaemoglobin?

This is a haemoglobin molecule that contains iron in the ferric (Fe^{3+}) state within its haem portion, as opposed to the normal ferrous (Fe^{2+}) state. It may be due to a congenital deficiency of reducing enzymes, or acquired through exposure to various chemicals such as the local anaesthetic agent prilocaine.

The molecule is less able to carry oxygen, and patients may appear cyanotic owing to the darker colour of methaemoglobin. It may be treated with the use of a reducing agent such as methylene blue.

How may ventilation be assessed?

Ventilation, which is a measure of the ability to blow off CO_2 adequately, may be measured and displayed visually by capnography. The end-tidal CO_2 is detected by a sensor placed at the exhaled stream of air. Owing to the relatively high solubility of CO_2, this is a good measure of the $PaCO_2$ when the ventilation and perfusion are well matched.

Capnography may also be used to assess airway patency, and in the detection of oesophageal intubation.

RENAL REPLACEMENT THERAPY

What types of renal replacement therapies are available?

These may be continuous or intermittent therapies

- *Haemodialysis:* continuous or intermittent
- *Haemofiltration:* a continuous form of renal replacement
- *Combination of dialysis and filtration:* continuous haemodiafiltration
- *Peritoneal dialysis*

What are the indications for commencing these?

The agreed indications for replacement therapy in renal failure are

- Fluid overload
- Hyperkalaemia of >6 mmol/l
- Acidosis with a pH of <7.2
- Urea of >30 mmol/l
- Those with chronic renal failure and a creatinine clearance of <10 ml/min
- Signs of encephalopathy

What are the basic features of haemodialysis and haemofiltration?

- *Haemodialysis:* the principle is that the blood interfaces the dialysis solution across a selectively permeable membrane that permits the passage of molecules of less than 5 kDa down a diffusion gradient. Unlike haemofiltration, it may be administered as either an intermittent or a continuous regimen

- *Haemofiltration:* this relies on the continuous convection of molecules across a membrane to which they are permeable. The fluid that is removed from the patient is replaced with a buffered physiological solution. Thus it is more effective in removing large volumes of fluid, but is not as effective as dialysis in clearing smaller molecules

When is intermittent haemodialysis used, and what are the basic components of the circuit?

This may be used several times per week in those with chronic renal failure and much less commonly used in the critically ill patient with acute renal failure. The essential components of the circuit are

- Vascular access point which may be through a central line or a surgical arteriovenous fistula for use in the long-term
- Extracorporeal circuit with an air trap and heparin pump to prevent air emboli and clotting in the circuit, respectively
- *Dialysis machine:* the dialysate solution passes through a dialyser cartridge that houses the diffusion membrane. Blood passes through, permitting diffusion across to the dialysate at the membrane interface
- The circuit is driven by a roller-pump

Give the most important complications of haemodialysis.

- *Dysequilibrium syndrome:* this follows sudden changes in the serum osmolality that occurs when molecules such as urea are filtered out. It can lead to cerebral oedema that usually presents with headaches, nausea and occasionally seizures

- *Hypotension* following a sudden reduction in the intravascular volume

- *Immune reactions* may occur when the extracorporeal circuit causes systemic complement cascade activation

- *Hypoxia:* as part of the systemic immune response leading to neutrophil aggregation in the lungs

- *Line sepsis*

- Loss of circuit connection leading to *air embolism or haemorrhage*

What types of continuous renal replacement therapies are there?

There are a number of continuous renal replacement modalities, depending on whether they rely on dialysis or filtration, and on the pattern of vascular connection

- *Continuous arteriovenous haemofiltration:* the flow is driven by the arteriovenous pressure difference

- *Continuous venovenous haemofiltration:* flow relies on roller pumps. This ensures that flow does not depend on the unstable arterial pressure of the critically ill patient. However, the patient must have good vascular access

- *Continuous arteriovenous or venovenous haemodialysis*

- *Haemodiafiltration:* a combination of both techniques that provides the best rate of urea clearance, and useful for hypercatabolic patients

How does peritoneal dialysis work?

Peritoneal dialysis is a slow form of continuous dialysis that relies on the peritoneum and its capillary network to act as the selectively permeable membrane. As with haemodialysis, solute flows down a diffusion gradient, and fluid flows by osmosis. The dialysate is introduced into the peritoneum by way of a Tenckhoff catheter and dwells within the abdomen for several hours before being drained off. This technique has been used in the intensive care setting, but has been superseded by other replacement therapies that are faster and more effective in removing urea and other solutes. However, it still has a place in the haemodynamically unstable patient, and the ambulating patient with chronic renal failure.

What is the classical infective complication? How is this recognised and treated?

The important infective complication is peritonitis that occurs following introduction of exogenous organisms. It may initially be recognised by the presence of a turbid effluent when the dialysate is drained, with >50 white cells per ml. It is caused

▼

by gram–positive organisms in 75% of cases, predominantly *Staphylococcus epidermidis* and *Staph. aureus*. Occasionally it is fungal. It may be managed by the addition of broad–spectrum antibiotics to the dialysate, such as cefuroxime and gentamicin.

RESPIRATORY ASSESSMENT

Which basic investigations may be used in assessing respiratory function?

The common respiratory investigations may be invasive or non-invasive.

Non-invasive

- *Peak flow rate:* a bedside measure of the airway resistance and respiratory muscle function

- *Sputum microscopy and culture*

- *Pulse oximetry:* measures arterial oxygen saturation and heart rate

- *Capnography:* measures end-tidal CO_2 as a marker of ventilatory function

- *Lung-function:*

  - *Spirometry:* to measure the lung volumes and forced expiration

  - *Gas transfer factor:* a measure of the diffusing capacity across the lung

- *Ventilation-perfusion scanning:* if pulmonary emboli are suspected

- *Echocardiography:* to assess pulmonary artery pressure and right heart function in cases of pulmonary hypertension and cor pulmonale

- *Imaging studies:* plain radiography, CT, MRI

Invasive

- *Arterial blood gas analysis:* direct measure of the oxygenation, ventilation and acid–base balance

- *Bronchoscopy:* may be flexible or rigid

- *Mediastinoscopy:* performed through an incision at the root of the neck, permitting biopsies of the regional lymph nodes

- *Lung biopsy:* may be performed as an open or thoracoscopic procedure, or CT-guided

What are the applications of fibreoptic bronchoscopy?

The applications may be both diagnostic and therapeutic

- Direct visualisation of the tracheobronchial tree in cases of obstruction
- Biopsy for cytology or histology: these may be obtained by direct sampling, or by use of the brush or washout technique. These applications are particularly important in cases of suspected malignancy or infection
- Aid in the removal of retained secretions: in these instances, it may even be performed through an endotracheal tube in the mechanically-ventilated patient
- Difficult intubation: including intubation with double-lumen endobronchial tubes
- As a therapeutic tool:
  - Removal of foreign bodies
  - Stenting of airways in cases of obstruction
  - Use of Nd Yag laser therapy for malignant obstruction

What is the advantage of rigid over flexible bronchoscopy?

Rigid bronchoscopy permits simultaneous instrumentation due to the wider lumen. This is useful in cases of foreign body removal and permitting suction when investigating massive haemoptysis.

Which of the lung volumes may be measured directly?

- Tidal volume: normally 7 ml/kg
- Vital capacity: normally 10–15 ml/kg
- Inspiratory capacity: inspiratory reserve volume + tidal volume

Define the functional residual capacity (FRC). What factors affect its volume?

The functional residual capacity is the volume of gas remaining in the lung at the end of a quiet expiration.

Factors that increase the FRC are
- Obstructive pulmonary diseases
- PEEP – which increases the intrathoracic pressure (i.e. makes it less negative)

Factors that reduce the FRC are
- Increased age and obesity
- Supine position
- Factors limiting lung expansion: pleural effusion, abdominal swelling and incision, thoracic incision, interstitial lung disease

What are the obstructive pulmonary diseases?
- Chronic bronchitis
- Emphysema
- Asthma
- Bronchiectasis

How do you differentiate obstructive from restrictive diseases on spirometry?

In cases of obstructive lung disease, there is an increase in the total lung capacity and residual volume due to air trapping. For restrictive diseases, there is a reduction of all of the lung volumes. The differences may be seen in the following diagrams:

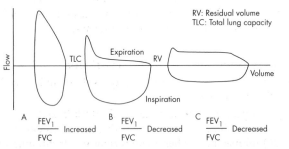

A = Restrictive lung disease   B = Obstructive lung disease   C = Upper airway obstruction

Flow volume loops of restrictive & obstructive defects, and in upper airway obstruction

Diagram from "Thoracic Surgery" 2nd ed, Edited by F. Griffith Pearson et al.
Published by Churchill Livingstone, ISBN 0443075956

RESPIRATORY FAILURE

What is the normal range for the PaO_2 and $PaCO_2$ in an individual breathing air at sea level?

The normal ranges are PaO_2 = 10.6–13.3 kPa, $PaCO_2$ = 4.7–6.0 kPa.

Why is ventilatory function best assessed by measuring the $PaCO_2$?

Alveolar ventilation (VA) is the volume of air that enters the alveoli each minute. Since all of the CO_2 produced by the body is excreted by exhalation during the process of alveolar ventilation, then

$PaCO_2 \times VA$ = amount of CO_2 exhaled in one minute.

Thus, $PaCO_2$ is proportional to $1/VA$.

It can be seen that measuring the CO_2 is key to assessing ventilation.

What is the definition of respiratory failure?

This is an acute or chronic failure of oxygenation, manifesting as a PaO_2 of <8 kPa owing to inadequate pulmonary gas exchange. It may also occur in the context of inadequate ventilation with CO_2 retention; CO_2 >6.7 kPa. The definition therefore depends on arterial blood gas analysis, but early recognition can be made on clinical suspicion.

How may respiratory failure be classified?

Respiratory failure is classified as types I, II and mixed, depending on the CO_2.

- *Type I (hypoxaemic) failure:* when PaO_2 <8 kPa, and normal or reduced $PaCO_2$. The pathology lies in either a V/Q mismatch, or when there is right to left shunting of blood (strictly speaking a 'pure' mismatch when the V/Q is 0). There is an initial elevation of the $PaCO_2$, stimulating the central chemoceptors that are sensitive to a local increase in the H^+ formed when CO_2 dissolves in the CSF. The resulting stimulation of ventilation blows off the CO_2 successfully, keeping the level in the normal range (or below it). Because of the flat-top of the sigmoidal O_2 dissociation curve, increasing the ventilation raises the PaO_2 very little. The outcome is therefore persisting hypoxaemia in the face of a normal or reduced $PaCO_2$ and tachypnoea

- *Type II (ventilatory) failure:* here, PaO_2 <8 kPa, $PaCO_2$ >6.7 kPa. It is characterised by alveolar hypoventilation leading to progressive hypercarbia. There is no compensatory increase in the ventilation, either because of respiratory 'apparatus' dysfunction, or because there is no compensation for a chronically elevated $PaCO_2$, as in COPD

- *Mixed defect:* the most common defect in the practical setting. A classical example is with any cause of type I defect where the patient develops exhaustion, producing a progressive and pre-terminal hypercarbia

Why should respiratory failure be classified?

The main purpose of classification lies in the practical use of oxygen as the therapeutic tool. In cases of chronic CO_2 retention, oxygen has to be used with caution (*see* 'Oxygen therapy').

Give some examples of the different causes of respiratory failure.

Type I

- *Shunt:* intracardiac, e.g. cyanotic congenital heart disease, Eisenmenger's syndrome

- *V/Q mismatch:*
  - Pneumonia (shunting may also occur at some lung units that are not being ventilated owing to inflammatory exudate)
  - Pulmonary embolism
  - Pulmonary oedema, e.g. cardiac failure, ARDS
  - Bronchiectasis, asthma

Type II
- *Cerebral lesion:* head injury, brainstem stroke, drug induced, e.g. barbiturates
- *Spinal lesion:* high cervical trauma, poliomyelitis
- *Peripheral nerve lesion:* motorneurone disease, Guillan–Barre syndrome
- *Neuromuscular junction lesion:* myasthenia gravis
- *Muscular lesion:* exhaustion, e.g. late acute severe asthma
- *Thoracic cage lesion:* flail chest injury with inefficient ventilation
- *Lung parenchymal lesion:* COPD with CO_2 retention, obstructive sleep apnoea

Outline the principles of management of respiratory failure.

The basic principles are
- Ensure adequate oxygenation: preferably humidified
- Ensure adequate ventilation: may need intubation and invasive respiratory support or CPAP
- Antibiotics if the underlying process is infective
- Management of other underlying causes, e.g. bronchodilators
- Others: airway suction, analgesics

RHABDOMYOLYSIS

What is myoglobin composed of and what is its function?

Myoglobin, a respiratory pigment found in cardiac and skeletal muscle, is composed of a single globin chain of 8 α helical regions with a single haem component. It acts as a ready source of oxygen for muscle during times of increased activity.

How does the oxygen dissociation curve for myoglobin differ from that of haemoglobin, and what accounts for this difference?

The shape of the dissociation curve for myoglobin is hyperbolic, as opposed to sigmoidal for haemoglobin. Unlike haemoglobin, CO_2 or pH does not affect the curve. The shape of the haemoglobin curve is a function of the interactions among the multiple globin chains and haem molecules. Myoglobin, consisting of only one globin chain and haem molecule does not exhibit these interactions.

What is rhabdomyolysis?

Rhabdomyolysis is a clinical syndrome caused by the release of potentially toxic muscle cell components into the circulation. It has many triggers including trauma, drugs, metabolic and congenital conditions.

What kinds of traumatic insult can trigger this off?

Trauma to muscle cell integrity may be caused by
- Blunt trauma to skeletal muscle, such as crush injury
- Prolonged immobilisation on a hard surface
- Massive burns
- Strenuous and prolonged spontaneous exercise
- Hypothermia
- Hyperthermia/hyperpyrexia
- Acute ischaemic and reperfusion injury

What complications may it lead to?

In the severest form, it may be complicated by

- *Acute renal failure:* may develop in up to 30% of those with rhabdomyolysis

- *Disseminated intravascular coagulation:* due to pathological activation of the coagulation cascade by the released muscle compounds

- *Compartment syndrome:* muscle injury may be associated with a rise in the intracompartmental pressure leading to worsening ischaemia

- Electrolyte disturbances

- *Hypovolaemia:* due to haemorrhage into the necrotic muscle. This may exacerbate the diminished renal function

List the associated electrolyte disturbances.

Disturbances include

- Hyperkalaemia with metabolic acidosis
- Hypocalcaemia
- Hyperphosphataemia
- Hyperuricaemia

What is the basic mechanism for the development of acute renal failure in rhabdomyolysis?

The exact mechanism is not fully understood but may involve ischaemic tubular injury caused by myoglobin and its breakdown products accumulating in the renal tubules.

How is the diagnosis of rhabdomyolysis confirmed?

- Elevated serum creatine kinase – up to five times the upper limit of normal. Elevations of the CK-MM isoenzyme is specific for skeletal muscle injury
- Elevated serum lactate dehydrogenase
- Elevated serum creatinine
- The presence of dark urine due to the presence of myoglobin. This is not always seen

R

- *myoglobinuria:* suggested by positive dipstick to blood in the absence of haemoglobinuria

All of these have to be taken in the context of a potential triggering factor.

What are the principles of management of a patient who has developed rhabdomyolysis following trauma?

The principle of therapy is largely supportive – managing complications and ensuring adequate renal function

- Ensure good hydration to support urine output with the use of i.v. crystalloid
- Diuretics such as mannitol may also be used for this end
- Alkalinising agent: sodium bicarbonate infusion has been used to limit myoglobin-induced tubular injury in the presence of acidic urine
- Management of associated electrolyte disturbances: particularly hyperkalaemia caused by the release of potassium by the injured muscle and exacerbated by metabolic acidosis. In the face of worsening renal function, dialysis or haemofiltration may have to be performed

What are the clinical features of compartment syndrome?

For compartment syndrome of the limbs:

- *Worsening pain:* which may be out of proportion to the injury
- *Paraesthesia:* especially loss of two point tactile discrimination

Clinical signs are

- Tense and swollen compartments
- Sensory loss
- Pain on passive stretching
- Loss of regional pulses: a late sign

▼

What levels of compartmental pressure may lead to compartment syndrome?

The first symptoms of pain and paraesthesia appear at compartmental pressures of 20–30 mmHg. Normal resting pressure is 0–8 mmHg.

What is the surgical management of compartment syndrome?

The primary treatment is decompression fasciotomy before the onset of necrosis and subsequent contracture. Some advocate a pressure of >30 mmHg as being the cut-off for fasciotomy, while others rely on the relationship of the compartmental pressure to the diastolic pressure.

SEPTIC SHOCK AND MULTI-ORGAN FAILURE

What is an endotoxin?

Endotoxin, a trigger of septic shock, is composed of the lipopolysaccharide derived from the cell walls of Gram negative bacteria. It has three components

- Lipid A: the lipid portion, and the source of much of the molecule's systemic effects
- Core polysaccharide
- Oligosaccharide side chains

What is the difference between bacteraemia and sepsis?

Bacteraemia refers to the presence of viable bacteria in the circulation. Sepsis is defined as the syndrome associated with the systemic response to infection. The latter is characterised by a systemic inflammatory response and diffuse tissue injury.

Define septic shock.

Septic shock is defined as the presence of sepsis with resulting hypotension or hypoperfusion, leading to organ dysfunction – despite adequate fluid replacement.

What particular feature distinguishes septic shock from cardiogenic or hypovolaemic shock?

The important feature of septic shock is the presence of a reduced systemic vascular resistance and an increased cardiac output. It has also been described as a 're-distributive' shock. The patient therefore has warm and vasodilated peripheries.

Cardiogenic or hypovolaemic shock is characterised by an increase in the systemic vascular resistance in response to a fall in the cardiac output. This manifests as cool peripheries, reflecting the reduced cardiac index (cardiac output per m^2 body surface area).

▼

What is the systemic inflammatory response syndrome (SIRS)?

The SIRS is the syndrome arising from the body's reaction to critical illness, such as overwhelming infection or trauma. Its presence is recognised and defined according to a number of clinical criteria

- Temperature of $>38°C$ or $<36°C$
- Heart rate of $>90/min$
- Respiratory rate of $>20/min$, or $PaCO_2$ of $<32\,mmHg$ (4.3 kPa)
- White cell count of $>12,000$ or $<4,000$ or greater than 10% immature forms

What triggers SIRS?

Triggers include

- Sepsis
- Multiple trauma
- Burns
- Acute pancreatitis

Thus many conditions other than sepsis may trigger these features. The concept of SIRS was introduced after it was shown that less than 50% of those who exhibited features of sepsis had positive blood cultures.

What are the basic pathophysiological events that lead to the development of SIRS?

The pathophysiology of this condition involves a progressive increase in the distribution of the inflammatory response in the body. The basic problem is a situation where the inflammatory response to the triggering event is excessive or poorly regulated. It has been described in terms of three phases

- *Phase I:* There is a local acute inflammatory response with the chemotaxis of neutrophil polymorphs and macrophages. Inflammatory mediators (such as cytokines and proteases) are released

- *Phase II:* These mediators are systemically distributed.
  Normally anti-inflammatory mediators such as IL-10
  ensure that the systemic response is limited

- *Phase III:* An overwhelming systemic cytokine 'storm' leads
  to the recognised systemic outcomes – pyrexia, tachycardia,
  peripheral vasodilatation and increased vascular
  permeability. There is a catabolic state with reduced tissue
  oxygen delivery despite increased oxygen demand

Name some important mediators that have been implicated in the development of SIRS.

- *IL-1:* induces pyrexia and leucocyte activation

- *IL-6:* involved in the acute phase response

- *IL-8:* involved in neutrophil chemotaxis

- *Platelet activating factor (PAF):* induces leucocyte activation
  and increased capillary permeability

- *Tumour necrosis factor alpha (TNF-α):* a pyrogen that
  stimulates leucocytes

Have you heard of the 'two-hit' hypothesis in the development of SIRS?

Yes, this is the observed finding that those with SIRS who are
recovering can have a rapid systemic response to a seemingly
trivial second insult, such as a urinary tract or line infection.
This may lead to a rapid and terminal deterioration in the
patient's state.

Define the multi-organ dysfunction syndrome (MODS).

The MODS is defined as the presence of altered and potentially reversible organ function in an acutely ill patient such
that homeostasis cannot be maintained without intervention.
By definition it affects two or more organs.

There are two types

- *Primary MODS:* the organ failure is directly attributable
  to the initial insult

▼

- *Secondary MODS:* the failure occurs as a result of the effects of SIRS. There may be a latent period between the initial event and the subsequent organ failure

Which organ systems may be involved in this process?

Any organ system may potentially be involved

- *Cardiovascular system:* there is vasodilatation with microcirculatory changes that increase the capillary permeability. This leads to a reduction of the systemic vascular resistance and maldistribution of blood flow. Initially there is a hyperdynamic state with increased cardiac output. Later, there is myocardial suppression

- *Lungs:* there is acute lung injury progressing to ARDS. This presents as pulmonary oedema, leading to V/Q mismatch and respiratory failure

- *Acute renal failure* due to acute tubular necrosis

- *Gut:* there is an ileus and intolerance to enteral feeding. Translocation of bacteria across the gut wall perpetuates sepsis

- *Liver* leading to deranged liver function

- *Coagulopathy* due to systemic activation of the coagulation cascade. This can lead to disseminated intravascular coagulation

- *Others:* such as bone marrow failure and neurological disturbances

Why may the gut fail in these situations?

There are a number of reasons

- The mucosa, which is very sensitive to ischaemia loses its integrity and function

- Exacerbated by maldistribution of blood flow

- Alterations in the number and type of gut flora

What is the mortality associated with organ failure?

- Mortality from renal failure is around 8%
- Mortality from renal failure + one other organ is around 70%
- Mortality from three failing organs is around 95%

What are the basic principles of management of any case of SIRS and MODS?

Management place a heavy emphasis on support of the failing organ systems

- *Surgical intervention:* sometimes required to reduce the infective load onto the circulation, e.g. drainage of pus

- *Circulatory support:* to maintain the cardiac index and oxygen delivery to the tissues with the use of i.v. fluids. Inotropes may be required, e.g. norepinephrine to increase the systemic vascular resistance. Monitoring therefore involves the insertion of a pulmonary artery flotation catheter

- *Ventilatory support* for the management of ARDS and respiratory failure. Note the risk of nosocomial pneumonia from intubation or aspiration

- *Renal support:* to ensure that the urine output is >0.5 ml/kg/h. Dopamine or a furosemide infusion may be required to support the failing kidney. Cardiac support helps maintain the renal perfusion pressure. Renal replacement therapies (haemofiltration, haemodialysis, and peritoneal dialysis) may also be required

- *Nutritional support:* may be enteral or parenteral. Enteral nutrition helps maintain mucosal integrity and reduce bacterial translocation

- Systemic antibiotics and infection surveillance. Initially, chemotherapy is empirical, but ultimately depends on culture results

SODIUM AND WATER BALANCE

What is the distribution of sodium in the body?

Sodium is the major extracellular cation of the body

- 50% is found in the extracellular fluid
- 45% is found in the bone
- 5% in the intracellular compartment

The vast majority (~70%) is found in the readily exchangeable form.

What are the major physiological roles of sodium?

Because of the content of sodium in the body, it exerts significant osmotic forces, and so important for internal water balance between the intra and extracellular compartments. It also has a role in determining external water balance and the extracellular fluid volume. The other important role of sodium is in generating the action potential of excitable cells.

What is the daily sodium requirement?

The daily requirement is about 1 mmol/kg/day.

What is the normal plasma concentration?

The normal is 135–145 mmol/l.

Give a simple classification of the causes of hyponatraemia.

- Water excess
  - *Increased intake:* polydipsia, iatrogenic, e.g. TURP syndrome, excess dextrose administration
  - *Retention of water:* SIADH
  - *Retention of water and salt:* nephrotic syndrome, cardiac and hepatic failure

- Water loss (with even greater sodium loss)
  - *Renal losses:* diuretics, Addison's disease, relief of chronic urinary obstruction
  - *Gut losses:* diarrhoea, vomiting
- Pseudohyponatraemia: in the presence of hyperlipidaemia

What is pseudohyponatraemia?

This is hyponatraemia that occurs as a peculiarity of the way in which the sodium concentration of the plasma is measured and expressed. In the presence of hyperlipidaemia or hyperproteiaemia, the sodium concentration may be falsely low if it is expressed as the total volume of plasma, and not just the aqueous phase (which it is normally confined to).

What is the TURP syndrome?

This is a syndrome of cardiovascular and neurological symptoms that occur following the use of hypotonic glycine-containing irrigation fluid with transurethral resection of the prostate.

The fluid and glycine are absorbed through the injured vessels to produce volume overload and hyponatraemia. It leads to bradycardia, blood pressure instability and confusion. In severe cases leads to convulsions and coma.

Which disease processes may trigger the syndrome of inappropriate ADH secretion (SIADH)?

SIADH may be triggered by the following

- *Lung pathology:*
  - Chest infection and lung abscess
  - Pulmonary tuberculosis
- *Malignancy:*
  - Small cell carcinoma of the lung
  - Brain tumours
  - Prostatic carcinoma

- *Intracranial pathology:*
  - Head injury
  - Meningitis
- Others, e.g. alcohol withdrawal

What does the term 'inappropriate' refer to in SIADH?

In this situation, there is an excessive and pathological retention of water in the absence of renal, adrenal or thyroid disease. The term 'inappropriate' refers to the fact that the urine osmolality is inappropriately high in relation to the plasma osmolality.

What are the clinical features of hyponatraemia?

The symptoms of hyponatraemia are due to water overload in brain cells. These can be non-specific, and include confusion, agitation, fits and a reduced level of consciousness. Other features depend on the underlying cause.

What are the causes of hypernatraemia?

The major causes may be classified as

- *Water loss:*
  - Diabetes insipidus
  - Insufficient intake or administration
  - Osmotic diuresis, e.g. hyperglycaemia
- *Excess sodium over water:*
  - Conn's or Cushing's syndrome
  - Excess hypertonic saline

What is diabetes insipidus?

This is a syndrome of polyuria, hypernatraemia with dehydration and compensatory polydipsia caused by an insensitivity to (nephrogenic form) or deficiency of (cranial form) ADH. Characteristically, fluid deprivation fails to concentrate the urine.

SPINAL INJURY

What is the incidence of spinal injuries in the UK?

The incidence is 15 per million per year.

What are the spinal cord syndromes associated with incomplete injuries?

There are three neurological syndromes associated with incomplete cord injuries

- *Central cord syndrome:* tends to occur in older individuals following hyperextension of the C-spine and compression of the cord against degenerative discs. Cord damage is centrally located

- *Anterior spinal cord syndrome:* the anterior aspect of the cord is injured, sparing the dorsal columns

- *Brown–Sequard syndrome:* following spinal hemisection

What are the patterns of deficit seen in each of the three syndromes?

- *Central cord syndrome:* motor weakness affects mainly the upper limbs. Sensory loss is usually less severe

- *Anterior spinal cord syndrome:* there is loss of motor function. There is also loss of pain and temperature sensation, but light touch, proprioception, and vibration sense are unaffected owing to preservation of the dorsal columns

- *Brown–Sequard Syndrome:* There is motor loss below the lesion, with contralateral loss of pain and temperature sensation. There is ipsilateral loss of dorsal column function

What deficits are seen in cases of complete injury?

The following deficits occur:

- *Motor deficit:* initial flaccid paralysis below the level of the lesion gives way to a spastic paralysis with increased tone

▼

and deep tendon reflexes due to loss of upper motorneurone input into the cord

- *Sensory deficit:* affecting the anterolateral and posterior columns. These therefore affect the somatic and visceral components to sensation

- *Autonomic deficit:* affecting the sympathetic and parasympathetic outputs of the cord

When would you suspect a spinal lesion in the unconscious trauma patient?

- Presence of multiple trauma, especially with head injuries
- Priapism in the male
- Paradoxical respiration due to diaphragmatic breathing when there is paralysis of the intercostal muscles. The level of the lesion in these cases is between C5 and C8
- Positive Babinski reflex: following loss of the upper motorneurone input. However, this is unreliable

Why may the trauma patient with a spinal injury exhibit bradycardia?

Bradycardia may occur with

- Loss of sympathetic outflow from the damaged cord
- Following a reflex increase in the cranial parasympathetic outflow due to airway suctioning
- The Cushing reflex due to elevated intracranial pressure if there is an associated head injury
- Pre-existing bradycardia due to cardiac disease or the use of drugs, such as β-adrenoceptor blockers

Why may spinal cord lesions lead to hypotension?

Hypotension may occur due to

- Loss of sympathetic outflow: there is loss of vasomotor tone leading to reduced systemic vascular resistance and, therefore, reduced arterial pressure
- Loss of sympathetic outflow can also produce bradycardia, which leads to a fall in the cardiac output and reduced arterial pressure

▼

- Occult blood loss, e.g. following blunt abdominal trauma with a visceral or vascular injury. Haemorrhage may be missed – it is easy to ascribe hypotension to the spinal injury alone

What are the dangers of autonomic dysfunction in these situations?

- Occult blood loss may be missed if there is hypotension, being erroneously ascribed to spinal trauma
- This may lead to overhydration during fluid resuscitation, leading to pulmonary oedema
- Hypotension reduces the cerebral perfusion pressure in the face of a head injury and rising intracranial pressure
- Bradycardia may be exacerbated when carrying out manoeuvres that stimulate the cranial parasympathetic outflow, e.g. intubation, airway suction, bladder distension. This may induce cardiac arrest. i.v. atropine must be at hand to reverse this process
- May lead to hypothermia due to loss of vasomotor control

What is 'spinal shock'?

This is a temporary state of flaccid paralysis that usually occurs very soon after a spinal injury, and may take 3–4 weeks to resolve. This is due to the loss of excitatory stimuli from supraspinal levels.

What drug has been used to minimise the extent of spinal injury following trauma?

High dose i.v. methylprednisolone has been used to limit secondary spinal injury from free radicals produced following trauma. For the most beneficial effect, it must be given within 8 h of trauma.

What does the immediate management of spinal injuries entail?

Immediate management involves prevention of secondary injury and management of potential complications associated with spinal injury

- C-spine immobilisation and careful handling of the patient can limit the damage if the spine has sustained an unstable injury
- Other injuries have to be sought, e.g. abdominal trauma or pulmonary injury (which can tip the patient into respiratory failure)
- Respiratory management with supplementary oxygen. If there is ventilatory failure, mechanical ventilation may be required
- Management of hypotension, this starts with exclusion of haemorrhage as the cause. Judicious use of i.v. fluids reduces the risk of pulmonary oedema. The arterial pressure may be supported with drugs such as atropine, α adrenoceptor agonists or the use of temporary cardiac pacing to increase the heart rate
- Prevention of hypothermia
- Prevention of gastric dilatation following the paralytic ileus of autonomic dysfunction. This involves nasogastric tube insertion. Gastric dilatation may splint the diaphragm, leading to respiratory failure
- Bladder catheterisation is required due to the risk of acute urinary retention with overflow incontinence
- DVT and gastric ulcer prophylaxis
- Surgical intervention may be required for unstable injuries, in the form of spinal fracture immobilisation and stabilisation

What are the important issues surrounding long-term management?

The most important aspect of long-term management is rehabilitation

- Prevention of decubitus ulcers

- Nutritional support for high spinal injuries in the form of percutaneous enteral feeding
- Bowel care with regular enemas and bulk-forming agents
- Bladder care with intermittent catheterisation
- Physiotherapy to help clear lung secretions (minitracheostomy may be required) and prevent limb contractures
- Psychological support and counselling as required

What is the difference between a Jefferson fracture and a hangman's fracture?

- *Jefferson fracture:* this is a burst fracture of C1 (atlas), best seen on the peg view. Seen as widening of the lateral masses and loss of congruity with the axis beneath. This is generally a stable injury
- *Hangman's fracture:* a fracture of C2 (axis) caused by hyperextension of the neck with the force of the occiput and the atlas bearing down on pedicle of C2

SYSTEMIC RESPONSE TO TRAUMA

Give some examples of stimuli that may activate the systemic stress response.

- Trauma resulting in pain and tissue injury
- Surgery
- Infection: endotoxin is a powerful stimulus
- Hypothermia
- Severe acid–base disturbances
- Acute hypoglycaemia

Which four physiological systems are involved in coordinating the systemic stress response?

- *Sympathetic nervous system:* producing changes in the cardiovascular endocrine and metabolic systems, e.g. promotes hyperglycaemia and activation of the renin–angiotensin–aldosterone (RAA) system

- *Endocrine system:* glucocorticoid release is stimulated by ACTH following the stress stimulus. Their plasma levels remain elevated for as long as the stimulus is present. Other hormones that are increased during the response are glucagon, thyroxine, growth hormone, histamine and endogenous opioids

- *Acute phase response:* with the release of cytokines, prostaglandins, leucotrienes and kinins

- *Microcirculatory system:* with changes in the vascular tone and permeability affecting tissue oxygen delivery. Vasoactive mediators such as nitric oxide, prostaglandins and platelet activating factor induce vasodilatation and increased capillary permeability

What are the main glucocorticoids in the body? Give some examples of some of their systemic effects.

The two main active glucocorticoids in the body are cortisol and corticosterone. Their effects are

- Metabolic:
  - *Glucose metabolism:* stimulation of gluconeogenesis and peripheral antagonism of insulin leads to hyperglycaemia and glucose intolerance
  - *Protein:* increased uptake of amino acids into the liver and promotion of protein catabolism in the peripheral tissues, such as muscle
  - *Lipid:* stimulation of lipolysis in adipose tissue
- Mineralocorticoid activity: promoting sodium and water retention with loss of potassium, all being mediated at the renal level
- Anti–inflammatory, immunosuppressive and anti–allergic actions
- Coordination of the stress response with a permissive effect on the actions of other hormones

Draw a diagram showing the change in the basal metabolic rate following a traumatic insult to the body.

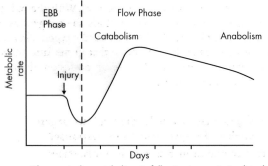

Changes in the metabolic rate following traumatic insult to the body

Diagram adapted from "Clinical Surgery in General"
Edited by Kirk, Mansfield & Cochrane, p 305
Published by Churchill Livingstone
ISBN 0443062196

What happens during the two phases of the metabolic response?

- *Ebb phase:* there is a reduction in the metabolic rate in the 24 h following the stimulus

- *Flow phase:* an increase in the metabolic rate, with generalised catabolism, negative nitrogen balance and glucose intolerance. The degree of metabolic increase depends on the type of initiating insult

Why is there a fall in the urine output immediately following a traumatic insult such as surgery? When does this resolve?

Following surgery, there is activation of the RAA system and increased release of antidiuretic hormone as part of the response. Thus, the urine output may remain low despite adequate volume replacement. It resolves usually in 24 h, but sodium retention may persist for several days longer.

Why may metabolic alkalosis develop and what effect does this have on oxygen delivery to the tissues?

The mineralocorticoid effects of cortisol and aldosterone promote sodium retention at the expense of potassium. Loss of potassium can lead to metabolic alkalosis. With the reduction of H^+ that defines metabolic alkalosis, the oxygen dissociation curve is shifted to the *left* (increased oxygen affinity), reducing tissue oxygen delivery. Note that in the latter stages of the response, if there is a fall in tissue perfusion, then the patient can become acidotic.

What changes may occur in the various organ systems during the systemic stress response?

- The cardiac output increases in the initial stages

- *Lungs:* hyperventilation leads to a respiratory alkalosis. In the latter stages, as part of the systemic inflammatory response, acute lung injury and ARDS may supervene

▼

- *Liver:* there is a reduction in the production of albumin
- *Clotting:* there is systemic activation of the coagulation cascade, which if severe enough, can lead to disseminated intravascular coagulation

TRACHEOSTOMY

Give some indications for tracheostomy.

- To maintain a patent airway in congenital defects of the face or upper airway, e.g. laryngotracheomalacia, laryngeal stenosis or cysts
- To maintain a patent airway following acquired pathologies, e.g. laryngeal tumors, post laryngectomy, diphtheria
- To maintain a patent airway in the emergency setting, e.g. laryngeal and upper airway trauma, laryngeal oedema, foreign body obstruction, inhalation injury
- To permit long-term positive pressure ventilation in those who are intubated for >2–3 weeks
- To facilitate airway suction
- To decrease the work of breathing and reduction of anatomic dead space, e.g. severe COPD, obstructive sleep apnoea

What kinds of tracheostomy do you know?

- *Open procedure performed by a surgeon:* There is dissection in the mid-line following division and ligation of the thyroid isthmus. A vertical incision is made between the 2nd, 3rd and 4th tracheal rings. Alternatively the trachea may have a window cut into it, or opened by lifting a flap of cartilage (Bjork flap). These two latter methods increase the risk of subsequent stenosis

- *Percutaneous tracheostomy:* A small skin crease incision is placed mid-way between the cricoid and sternal notch. A guide wire is advanced through a 14G cannula that has been passed through the incision. Dilators of increasing diameter are sequentially passed through to widen the aperture. Alternatively, dilating forceps widen the tracheostomy, so that the tube can be inserted into the correct position. Fibreoptic bronchoscopy can be used to aid placement

- *Translaryngeal tracheostomy:* A guide wire is passed into the mouth via a cannula that pierces the trachea. The cuffed tube is passed into the mouth and fed over the wire and into the trachea, part exiting through the anterior tracheal wall

- *Minitracheostomy:* A 4 mm-diameter-uncuffed tube is passed through the median cricothyroid ligament under local anaesthetic. It permits regular tracheal suction and high-flow jet ventilation in the emergency setting

What problems can arise if the incision is too high or too low?

If incision is placed too high, it can lead to sub-glottic stenosis, if placed too low, it can lead to a tracheo–inominate fistula.

What are the advantages of a percutaneous technique?

- Does not require the presence of a surgeon
- Can be carried out in the ITU, avoiding the operating room
- More rapid, and less traumatic than the open method

How do tracheostomies in children differ from those in adults?

- In children, low placement should be avoided due to the high risk of injury to the left brachio-cephalic vein that may run above the sternal notch
- In children, access to the tracheal lumen should be performed through a vertical slit. Removal of cartilage leads to tracheal stenosis
- Cuffed tubes should generally be avoided in children because of the risk of mucosal ulceration and tracheal stenosis
- Under the age of 12, percutaneous tracheostomy should be avoided due to the risk of oesophageal injury

What types of tracheostomy tubes are there?

A number of different types of tubes exist

- Metal or plastic
- Cuffed or uncuffed. Cuffed reduces the risk of aspiration
- Fenestrated or unfenestrated: The fenestration permits speech

What are the complications of tracheostomies?

Complications may be in the early or late stages:

- Early:
  - Bleeding: Especially from the stump of the thyroid isthmus or anterior jugular vessels. Adrenaline-soaked swabs can be used to control minor ooze
  - Injury to surrounding structures, e.g. oesophageal perforation, injury to recurrent laryngeal nerves, pleural reflections, brachiocephalic vein, subcutaneous emphysema
  - Tube displacement and inadvertent extubation
  - Blockage by encrusted secretions
- Mid-term:
  - Infection: Ranging from superficial wound problems to tracheitis
  - Tracheo-inominate fistula if erosion occurs into this local structure. Presents as a severe haemorrhage
- Late:
  - Mucosal ulceration and tracheal stenosis

Once in place, how are tracheostomy tubes cared for?

Care of the tube is top-priority

- The tube is secured in place
- Broad-spectrum antibiotics are commenced for a few days
- Humidified oxygen is given for the first few days
- The cuffed tube is changed to an uncuffed tube after several days

T

- The tube requires regular cleaning – sometimes even twice per day to prevent the build-up of encrusted secretions. This involves the removal of the inner tube and cleaning in a solution such as hydrogen peroxide
- Emergency equipment should always be at the ready – such as suction devices, replacement tubes and tracheal dilators

TRANSFER OF THE CRITICALLY ILL

What is meant by primary and secondary transfer?

- Primary transfer is the movement of the patient from the scene of trauma to the site of hospital care. It is managed and organised by the pre-hospital team that usually comprises of paramedics

- Secondary transfer involves the movement of the patient between hospitals, where they can receive specialist investigations and treatments, e.g. neurosurgical units for the head–injured

What types of transportation may be used to transfer the critically ill?

The principle forms of transport employed are

- *Ground ambulance:* providing door to door transport, but at the cost of reduced speed

- *Air ambulance:* either as a helicopter or aeroplane. This may include the added hazard of transfer at high altitude. Also requires a designated landing site

- *By water:* not routinely employed

What are the dangers of a high altitude transfer?

There are two main dangers

- *Hypoxia:* due to a reduction in the atmospheric pressure associated with an increasing altitude. This is not usually a problem since the critically ill should receive supplemental oxygen from an cylinder

- *Gaseous expansion:* This leads to rapid tension of a simple pneumothorax if it goes unrecognised. For this reason bilateral chest drains may be required prior to transfer in those with suspected chest injuries. Also can lead to worsening bowel distension in those with bowel obstruction

Which three groups of people are the most important as far as communication is concerned?

The three most important groups of people that need to be communicated with closely are

- The person who is to be transferred: if they are conscious
- The receiving unit
- The relatives of the patient

What types of equipment should be available during transfer?

- Oxygen cylinders
- Portable mechanical ventilator
- Airway equipment: endotracheal tubes, airway adjuncts
- Suction device
- i.v. access
- i.v. fluids
- Cardiac defibrillator with a back-up power source
- Drugs: cardiac, respiratory, resuscitation and anaesthetic
- Monitoring equipment: cardiac and respiratory monitoring devices

How is the patient prepared prior to transfer?

- Securing haemodynamic stability
- Respiratory stability: the portable ventilator should meet the needs of the patient. If there is a chest drain *in situ*, then its position must be checked and the under-water seal drain must be well placed
- Body temperature must be stabilised, with the prevention of hypothermia
- Requirements for sedation muscle relaxation and analgesia must be seen to

TUBE THORACOSTOMY (CHEST DRAIN)

What is the purpose of a chest drain?

This is both a diagnostic and therapeutic procedure that enables drainage of air and fluid (effusion, blood, pus, and lymph) from the pleural space, thereby enabling re-expansion of the lung.

Which sizes of chest drains are available?

Sizes 20–32 French gauge (F) may be used. Generally for adults 28F is adequate for most uses. To prevent clot obstruction when draining blood, size 32F is used. The French Gauge refers to the external circumference in millimeters, being roughly three times the external diameter.

Outline the steps for insertion.

The following steps are involved in insertion at the bedside

- The patient is fully informed as to why the drain is required, reassured, and talked through the steps
- Clinical examination of the patient and inspection of the chest radiograph confirm the side of insertion
- The patient is positioned. This may be supine with the arm abducted over the site of insertion. Alternatively, the patient may be seated, leaning forward on to a table with the arms outstretched
- The skin over the site of insertion is cleaned with povidone-iodine solution, and draped with a sterile towel
- The 5th intercostal space in the mid-axillary line is identified by palpation of the ribs
- A wheal is raised over this site with a small amount of local anaesthetic, such as 1 or 2% lignocaine with an orange needle. This is changed to a larger-bore green needle, and advanced more deeply
- To prevent injury to the neurovascular bundle that runs in the subcostal groove, the needle is advanced over the top

of the rib below, infiltrating all the while with local anaesthetic

- To confirm entry into the pleural space at the deeper levels, the plunger is withdrawn to obtain fluid or air
- Once adequate anaesthesia has been achieved, a 1–1.5 cm incision is made with a scalpel. This is best performed with a single, controlled stab with a size 11 blade
- Blunt dissection down to the pleura is performed using the little finger and Robert's forceps. Once the parietal pleura is punctured, the finger is swept inside to clear any adhesions and widen the tract
- The drain is guided into the intercostal space while the tip is held with the Robert's forceps. This is performed without the use of the trocar
- To drain air the tip is guided apically, to drain fluid it is guided basally
- The drain is secured by a silk or nylon purse-string suture, and a clean dressing placed over the thoracostomy site

What essential procedures need to take place following insertion?

Following insertion, the following must take place

- Attachment to an under-water seal drain system, with or without suction
- A chest radiograph is taken to ensure accurate positioning, and confirm lung re-expansion
- Analgesia is given to the patient

What are the indications for removal of the drain?

Indications include

- The drain is no longer functioning
- Full expansion of the lung, as seen on the chest radiograph
- Air and fluid have ceased to drain. For example, no further respiratory swing on the drain, cessation of

▼

bubbling seen when suction is applied (suggesting that a parenchymal air-leak has sealed)

What determines an adequate underwater-seal drain system?

For an underwater-seal system to be competent, it must have certain properties

- The drain bottle should be held below the level of the patient at all times
- To minimise resistance, the chest tube should be sufficiently wide
- The end of the drainage tube must not be more than 5 cm below the level of the water in the bottle, or the resistance encountered will prevent air from escaping the chest tube

Why is bupivicaine not used as a local anaesthetic during bedside drain insertion?

Bupivicaine is an amide local anaesthetic, which although has a longer duration of action than lignocaine, has a slower onset of action. For this reason, it is not a suitable agent when being used on the conscious patient.